CHRONIC LOW BACK PAIN

Chronic Low Back Pain

Editors

Michael Stanton-Hicks, M.B.B.S., F.F.A.R.C.S.
Chairman
Department of Anaesthesia
University of Massachusetts Medical Center
Worcester, Massachusetts

Robert A. Boas, M.B., CH.B., F.F.A.R.A.C.S.
Associate Professor
Department of Pharmacology and Clinical Pharmacology
University of Auckland School of Medicine
Auckland, New Zealand

Raven Press ■ New York

Raven Press, 1140 Avenue of the Americas, New York, New York 10036

Great care has been taken to maintain the accuracy of the information contained in the volume. However, Raven Press cannot be held responsible for errors or for any consequences arising from the use of the information contained herein.

Library of Congress Cataloging in Publication Data
Main entry under title:

Chronic low back pain.

Includes bibliographical references and index.
1. Backache.   2. Backache—Treatment.   I. Stanton-Hicks, Michael d'A.   II. Boas, Robert A.   III. Title: Low back pain. [DNLM: 1. Backache. WE 755 C557]
RD768.C5   617'.56   82–339
ISBN 0–89004–598–4

Preface

The longtime back sufferer and his artful therapist have been witnesses to many changes in therapeutic emphasis in recent years, with some treatments bordering on cultist and others proclaiming scientific validity—all of them seeking to resolve our greatest disabling complaint of low back pain. A renewed surge of interest in nonmedical practices and growth of singular therapy techniques attest to both the failure of conventional medicine to solve this problem and the public demand for an alternative. By a similar default, the entry of many newer disciplines into the field of back pain management has come about in an attempt to seek a greater comprehension of the problems involved and how they can be met. As yet, the progress has been limited, both with respect to cause and cure, though some advances have certainly been made.

The authors in this volume foster a wider understanding of all aspects of low back pain. This understanding involves the poorly recognized aspects of natural history, etiology, psychosocial and functional components of pain and disease as well as the more conventional aspects of therapy. The therapeutic emphasis is on newer and better conservative management and on a more profound critical attitude among practitioners. In addition, the authors provide a consensus as to how best to attain a quick, safe, and effective functional restoration for the vast majority of patients with low back pain.

Having experienced the high standard of presentations and enthusiasm for the philosophies and techniques espoused, we believe that the collection of papers in this volume will help others who similarly seek both direction and technique in their approach to patient care of low back pain. The papers are therefore written with a view to present each author's understanding and experience rather than a review of the subject. Our hope is that those practitioners who desire a greater understanding and a larger role in the care of their patients with back pain will better utilize the many therapies available to them and will be better able to assist the long-term patients whose expectations and frustrations remain unbounded.

Michael Stanton-Hicks
Robert A. Boas

Contents

Contributors

David J. Berg, D.O.
Chief, Special Procedures Section
Department of Radiology
Phoenix General Hospital
Phoenix, Arizona 85015

Robert A. Boas, M.B., CH.B., F.F.A.R.A.C.S.
Associate Professor in Anaesthetics
Department of Pharmacology and Clinical Pharmacology
University of Auckland School of Medicine
Auckland, New Zealand

Rene Cailliet, M.D.
Professor and Chairman
Department of Rehabilitative Medicine
University of Southern California School of Medicine
Los Angeles, California 90033

John J. Calabro, M.D., F.A.C.P.
Director of Rheumatology
Saint Vincent Hospital
Professor of Medicine and Pediatrics
University of Massachusetts Medical School
Worcester, Massachusetts 01604

Harold Carron, M.D.
Director Emeritus
Pain Clinic
Department of Anesthesiology
University of Virginia Medical Center
Charlottesville, Virginia 22908

Linda Czerniawski, R.P.T.
Assistant Director of Physical Therapy
University of Massachusetts Medical Center
Worcester, Massachusetts 01604

Thomas G. Kantor, M.D.
Professor of Clinical Medicine
Department of Medicine
New York University School of Medicine
New York, New York, 10016

W. Monroe Keyserling, Ph.D.
Assistant Professor
Department of Environmental Health Sciences
Harvard School of Public Health
Boston, Massachusetts 22115

John D. Loeser, M.D.
Professor of Neurological Surgery
Assistant Dean for Curriculum
University of Washington School of Medicine
Seattle, Washington 98195

James E. McLennan, M.D.
Assistant Professor of Neurosurgery
Pain Consultant, Pain Control Center
University of Cincinnati Medical Center
Cincinnati, Ohio 45267

Alf Nachemson, M.D.
Chairman and Professor
Department of Orthopaedic Surgery
Sahlgren Hospital
Göteborg, Sweden

Lawrence E. Peterson, Ph.D.
Assistant Professor of Anesthesiology
and Psychiatry
Pain Control Unit
University of Massachusetts Medical
School
Director, Clinical Psychology
Training
Chief Psychologist
Department of Psychology
Worcester State Hospital
Worcester, Massachusetts 01605

James C. Phero, M.D.
Assistant Professor of Anesthesia
Pain Consultant, Pain Control Center
University of Cincinnati Medical
Center
Cincinnati, Ohio 45267

P. Prithvi Raj, M.D.
Professor of Anesthesia
Director, Pain Control Center
University of Cincinnati Medical
Center
Cincinnati, Ohio 45267

James L. Schaepe, M.D.
Medical Director
The Norton Company
Worcester, Massachusetts 01606

J. A. Skeleton, Ph.D.
Assistant Professor
Department of Psychology
Dickinson College
Carlisle, Pennsylvania 17013

Gerald G. Steinberg, M.D.
Associate Professor of Orthopedic
Surgery
University of Massachusetts Medical
Center
Worcester, Massachusetts 01605

Ann Gill Taylor, R.N., Ed.D.
Associate Professor of Nursing
Director
Medical-Surgical Nursing Major,
Graduate Program
School of Nursing
University of Virginia
Charlottesville, Virginia 22908

Timothy C. Toomey, Ph.D.
Clinical Associate Professor
of Psychology
Pain Clinic
Dental Research Unit
University of North Carolina
Dental School
Chapel Hill, North Carolina 27514

Harold A. Wilkinson, M.D., Ph.D.
Chairman and Professor
Neurosurgery Department
University of Massachusetts Medical
Center
Worcester, Massachusetts 01605

Chronic Low Back Pain, edited by
M. Stanton-Hicks and Robert Boas.
Raven Press, New York © 1982.

Epidemiology of Low Back Pain

Gerald G. Steinberg

*Department of Orthopedics, University of Massachusetts Medical Center,
Worcester, Massachusetts 01605*

It is difficult to approach the epidemiology of back pain as we would approach the epidemiology of any other medical problem. Epidemiology is concerned with the incidence and prevalence of a disease and the determinants of disease prevalence. Back pain is not a disease but, in fact, is a final common pathway complaint for a number of different disease states. In the international classification of diseases, there are at least thirty different entries that describe conditions that primarily cause back pain and many others in which back pain can be part of the clinical presentation (51). Consequently, one is really looking at the epidemiology of a number of different pathologic conditions, all of which cause back pain. This must be kept in mind when one reviews the statistics that relate to back pain. In addition, since the complaint of back pain is so subjective, the complaint itself is difficult to define. Does one study all back pain, no matter how trivial or short-lived? Does one include only those that require medical attention? How does one account for patients who have much pain and complain little versus patients who have little pain and complain much? The task is difficult and, although it is important to look at the epidemiology of back pain, it is almost impossible to validate its frequency completely accurately and objectively.

Within these limitations much data has been gathered concerning the epidemiology of back pain. However, reviewing these studies is a little bit like eating popovers—one has to bite into and chew up a lot of hot air in order to get something solid to swallow. In this chapter, we shall try to concentrate on the edibles. A careful and critical review of the available studies will provide us with an approximation of the frequency of back pain, an understanding of its natural history, an appreciation of some of the determinants of the prevalence of back pain, and finally, an estimate of the size of the problem created by the person who is of greatest concern, the chronic back pain sufferer.

FREQUENCY OF LOW BACK PAIN

Back pain occurs in 50 to 80% of the population of developed industrial societies (15,16,18,19,29). There have been several significant studies done over the last 20 years on the frequency of low back pain (6,15,16,18,29). The range of frequency reported in these studies is wide, from 47 to 79%. Such a wide range may appear

1

extreme and deserves comment. These statistics on the general prevalence of back pain have to be obtained through interview techniques. They can be substantiated by examination, X-rays, and disability records, but the interview itself is the most important tool in indicating the frequency with which this condition is affecting a particular population. Thus the generated data become more or less accurate depending upon the nature of the interview process, the questions asked, the recall of the person interviewed, etc. This explanation, in large part, accounts for the variability in the reported frequencies. When the published data are reviewed on the basis of these criteria, it appears that the most thorough studies come from Sweden, and the real frequency of back pain is in the upper half of this range.

In 1969, Horal (16) published his study of the clinical appearance of low back disorders in Götenborg, Sweden. He looked at two groups of people. One group, which he called the "sick-listed" group, had been out of work for 1 week during the study year because of back pain. A second group of matched controls had not been sick-listed during the study year and, in addition, had not been sick-listed because of back pain for 12 years prior to the study. In the control group, Horal noted a 66.5% frequency of back pain, a frequency that is probably lower than the real prevalence of back pain in that population because those individuals with the most severe symptoms, i.e., the sick-listed indivduals, were excluded from the control group.

In 1954, Hult (18) studied a group of industrial and forest workers and showed a 79% frequency of low back pain. In a subsequent study, published that same year, 1,200 light and heavy industry workers were reviewed and a frequency of 60% of low back pain was noted in a group of male workers, age 25 through 59.

These figures indicate the frequency with which back pain is noted to have occurred at some time during the lives of individuals in these populations. These figures are high because they represent lifetime occurrence. The incidence, or frequency of occurrence, over a specific period of time is, of course, much lower and depends upon the length of time being considered. This type of data has also been gathered. In 1969, Lawrence (29) published a study from Great Britain that showed a 15% incidence of back pain at the time of interview. In Horal's study (16), a much higher incidence of symptoms at the time of interview—a rate of 39%—was noted, whereas in a study by Partridge et al. (38), 11% of those questioned were having symptoms at the time of interview and 34% reported symptoms over the prior year. In 1973, Nagi et al (36) reported that 18% of those interviewed in a household survey in the state of Ohio claimed that they had "often been bothered by back pain" in the recent past, and Magora (35) published data from Israel that showed a 14% yearly incidence of back pain.

In summary, based on the available data, back pain as a general condition affects nearly 75% of the population of most industrial societies. In addition, the reported incidence is such that at least 10 to 15% of these populations appears to be affected by back pain yearly.

NATURAL HISTORY OF LOW BACK PAIN

The obvious question to ask at this point is, what happens to these millions of back pain sufferers? What is the natural history of this condition? Obviously, these people don't all seek medical attention in our offices and clinics or we would be overrun by their numbers.

To begin with, it is clear that low back pain is usually a self-limited condition. Dixon (8) demonstrated in statistics from Great Britain that 90% of all episodes of back pain recover without a physician's consultation. This is probably because most episodes of back pain are mild. In Horal's study (16), only 3% of those with mild symptoms sought medical attention. Even for those who seek medical attention, remission is the rule. From Fry's statistics (10), 40 to 50% of those attending clinic showed improvement within 1 week and 90% improved within 8 weeks. Most of the published data is in agreement with this, with an 80 to 90% improvement within 2 months regardless of treatment (7,16,18). Additional data indicates that recovery is rapid and complete enough that for a given episode seen by a general practitioner, 97% of patients avoid hospitalization and 99.5% avoid surgery (5,53). Furthermore, few patients suffer for a long period. In Horal's study (16), only 2.4% of controls and 4% of sick-listed patients suffered for more than 6 months with any given episode. Similarly, in Hult's study (18), there was only a 4% frequency of disability of more than 6 months' duration.

At first glance, we might look at the figures above and feel that we are "off the hook." Although the problem is ubiquitous, it appears to be self-limited. The fact is, however, that we are not off the hook for two reasons. First, the general prevalence rate is so high that even a low percentage of persistent complainers creates a large number of chronic back pain sufferers. Second, although back pain is characterized by a high spontaneous remission rate, it is also characterized by a high recurrence rate. Horal noted recurrence in 90% of the patients who were "sick-listed" and 67% of the symptomatic controls (16). Other studies demonstrate a similarly high recurrence rate, in the 70 to 80% range (6,15). In addition, it is clear that repeat episodes last longer and are more severe than the initial attack (16).

In summary then, it appears that although back pain is a ubiquitous problem, most episodes are mild and recover without physician consultation. Even for individuals who consult a physician, there is a 95% rate for remissions that occur within 6 months. However, although a high remission rate is characteristic, so too is a high recurrence rate. It is this high recurrence rate combined with the relatively small percentage but large absolute number of people suffering beyond 6 months that creates an enormous group of people who constitute the chronic and recurrent back pain sufferers.

From the statistics just reviewed, there should be an estimated several million people suffering from chronic back pain in this country. This estimate is, in fact, borne out by observed data that will be presented below.

DETERMINANTS OF THE PREVALENCE OF BACK PAIN

At this point, one should look to see what factors, if any, have a significant effect on the general prevalence of back pain.

Sex

The first question one might ask is whether men or women have more back pain. It should be noted that the data in this area are in conflict. There is some evidence to suggest that women may be more prone to back pain when exposed to heavy work (32,36) and that men may be more prone to back pain arising from a herniated lumbar disk (21). However, most large studies fail to show any clear evidence that sex has a significant effect on the general frequency of back pain (15,16,29,38).

Age

Age is of definite importance; there is a significant age dependency when one considers low back pain. The table summarizes data from four major studies that evaluate the frequency of back pain per decade of age. The peak in each study is indicated in heavy print. Thus, in Horal's study the peak frequency was in the fifth decade (16); in the studies by Hult (18), Lawrence (29), and Hirsch et al (15), it was in the sixth decade. A graph of the frequencies per decade of age, which is derived by averaging the results from the four studies, clearly shows that the frequency of low back pain peaks towards the end of the fifth and the early part of the sixth decade of age and seems to taper off after that (Fig. 1). In terms of age of onset, the third decade is when back pain becomes a significant problem (16,18). The most usual time for back trouble to begin is between the ages of 20 and 30. Thus, a second graph created by averaging the data from Hult's and Horal's studies, shows a clear peak for age of onset in the third decade, with the fourth

TABLE. 1. *Percent of population with low back pain complaints for each age group*

Study (ref. no.)	Age in decades (years)				
	3rd (20–29)	4th (30–39)	5th (40–49)	6th (50–59)	7th (60–69)
Horal (16)	52	65	79[a]	66	63
Hult (18)	34[b]	49	65	71[a]	
Lawrence (29)	14[c]	47	68	85[a]	57
Hirsch et al. (15)	18[c]	44	60	68[a]	68
Average percent	30	51	68	73	63

[a]Number represents peak frequency of patients with back complaints in this study.
[b]Age group is 25 to 29 years.
[c]Age group is below 24 years.

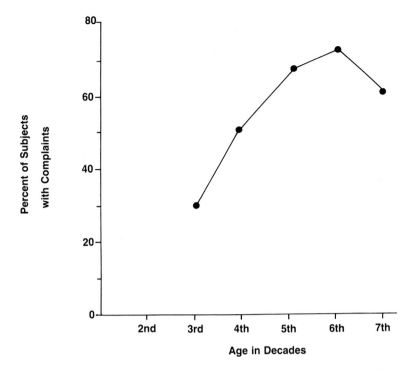

Fig. 1. For each decade of age, the percent of subjects with past or present back pain complaints is shown. The percent values for each decade are calculated by averaging the data from studies by Hirsch et al. (15), Horal (16), Hult (18), and Lawrence (29).

decade close behind (Fig. 2). These data further suggest that by age 45 most people who develop back pain will have had their first episode. Combining the figures for age of onset with figures for peak incidence, the greater majority of back pain sufferers can be placed between the ages of 25 and 55.

X-RAY APPEARANCE

In general, the X-ray appearance of the lumbar spine does not correlate with the complaint of acute back pain. Although over 90% of people who have suffered from lumbar pain show some type of X-ray abnormality, X-rays of the lumbar spines of people not complaining of back pain show a similar high rate of various abnormalities (16). The fact is that most of these X-ray abnormalities are not associated with back pain. Lumbar facet asymmetry, spina bifida occulta, hyper-lordosis, mild scoliosis, lumbarization or sacralization of the lumbar spine do not show statistically significant correlation with low back pain (16,18). On the other hand, spondylolisthesis and, to a lesser extent, disk degeneration do appear to correlate with low back pain. The statistics in regard to spondylolisthesis are fairly clear, and most studies show a uniformly high rate of back pain in people with this

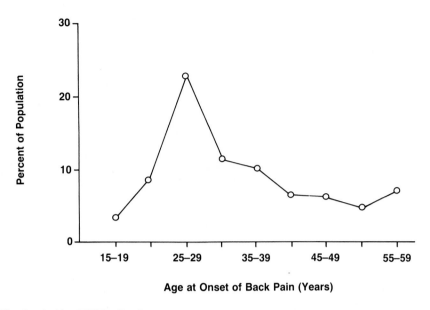

Fig. 2. Incidence of back pain onset per age group is shown for a population comprised of subjects who have experienced an episode of back pain. Data are taken from studies by Horal (16) and Hult (18).

condition (16,18). The situation in regard to disk generation is a bit more complicated. The frequency and degree of disk degeneration are directly correlated with the subject's age. This was clearly established in the classic autopsy studies of Schmorl and Junghanns (40) on the problem of degenerative disk disease. These studies demonstrated that by the end of the fourth decade 50% of the population shows signs of degenerative changes in the spine and that the prevalence rises sharply, approaching 100% in later decades. The percentages are similar for men and women, although the rate of degeneration with age is slightly higher in men in the fourth and fifth decades. X-ray studies of degenerative changes in the spine have not shown quite as high an absolute percentage of abnormality as these autopsy studies. This is to be expected since the X-ray is not as sensitive a tool as the autopsy for noting degenerative changes in the spine. The figures, however, are not that different. Thus, Hult, who evaluated the frequency of the disk degeneration as noted on X-ray in different age groups, showed that by the end of the fourth decade, approximately 40% of the population showed signs of degenerative changes and that the prevalence approached 90% in later decades (18). These figures represent an analysis of the entire population. In Hult's analysis of populations with and without back pain, he did show that in essentially all age groups the frequency of disk degeneration was higher in those individuals who had had an episode of back pain. The difference, however, was slight and consequently not statistically significant enough that one could consider the X-ray finding of disk degeneration a significant determinant of back pain in that population. However, Hult looked further into the data and when he separated patients with evidence of pronounced degenerative changes on X-ray, he did find a significant increase in the frequency of back pain in the individuals with such changes, especially in the older age groups. This correlation of back pain with degenerative changes was not only seen in Hult's work, but also in the work of Horal and Lawrence (16,29). It should be emphasized here that this correlation is with previous episodes of pain, not with current episodes of pain.

In summary of the findings of X-ray changes, only spondylolisthesis is a significant determinant of back pain in the individual subject. Disk degeneration shows a weaker correlation with previous episodes of pain. This correlation only appears to be significant in older subjects with moderate or severe changes at 1 or 2 levels of the lumbar spine. Changes of this type in the older individual probably do indicate that the person has a higher chance of having had back pain in the past and perhaps developing back pain in the future.

OCCUPATION

There is much evidence showing some increase in low back symptoms in people who do heavy versus light work (1,11,12,18,19,28,29,32,33,36). For instance, Hult (18), in a comparative study of 471 retail, light industry, and sedentary workers versus 666 construction, food handling, and other heavy industry workers, showed that the frequency of low back pain was 52% in the group that did lighter work versus 64% in the heavy work group (18). This degree of difference has been noted in many other studies. It is not a large difference and consequently is not great enough to suggest that heavy work per se is significant as a determinant of back pain. However, if one looks more closely, an additional factor appears. If one considers only those people suffering from severe back pain, a much larger difference is noted. Once again, looking at Hult's data as an example, the group that did lighter work had a 6.8% prevalence of severe back pain whereas the group doing heavier work had a 10.6% prevalence. This change in frequency represented a 50% increase from the light to the heavy work group and is certainly significant. The situation in regard to occupational stress and back pain is thus similar to what we found in regard to disk degeneration. The significant correlation was not found in the general statistics but rather in the group with severe changes and severe symptoms. It should be added that as far as work disability is concerned, i.e., inability to work as opposed to the prevalence of the problem, the data clearly show a higher prevalence of sick days in those that do heavy work (18). This doesn't have so much to do with a real difference in the frequency of the problem but rather with the fact that if one's back hurts, it is much harder to do a job that involves heavy work. In addition, it has to be recognized that persons who think of their work as physically demanding have a higher incidence of back pain. This has been well substantiated by Magora (33). There are other significant factors in regard to occupation that deserve mention. Most authors agree that there is increased prevalence of back pain in those who have prolonged postural stress (34). For example, there is a higher and earlier prevalence of back pain in motor vehicle drivers who sit for long periods of time (20,22,32). This would include truck and bus drivers. There is a higher prevalence of back pain in miners who perform heavy work in stooped positions and where the footing is frequently poor (25,28,30). Back pain is also more prevalent in nurses who do awkward episodic lifting (9,32). Occupational factors, however, are quite complex and lifting heavy objects is not necessarily the predisposing element in back pain. Kelsey (21) was unable to demonstrate an increased risk for "disk herniation" for individuals whose jobs involved lifting, pulling, pushing, or carrying. Likewise, Rowe's industrial studies (39) did not show a preponderance of heavy workers with "discogenic" back pain. In Hult's study (18), the incidence of back pain and disk degeneration in a group of weightlifters was compared with individuals who did light and heavy work. In the older age groups, the weightlifters actually had a lower incidence of symptoms and a lower prevalence of disk degeneration on X-ray. In the final analysis, it is not work specifically that leads to back pain, but rather one's fitness for the performance of a certain type of work that is the significant determinant.

There are many other factors that have been considered in exploring the epidemiology of back pain. Some of these associations are interesting and plausible. Kelsey et al (23) showed an increased incidence of back pain in those who live in suburban versus urban environments; this is probably related to the amount of time that is spent driving. Certain studies relate the onset of back pain to a specific accident or heavy lifting episode. From analysis of industrial data, the percentage of individuals that recall this type of relationship is high, as one would expect (11,27,44). In one study, over 85% of individuals who presented with back pain related it to a specific incident (27). However, in the more general studies, this association is seen with lesser degrees of frequency (16). In Hult's study (18), only 30 to 40% of the cases were associated with a specific accident or lifting episode. Rowe (39) found that trauma was "rarely involved" in a precipitation of discogenic backache.

As noted, much of the epidemiologic research is interesting and plausible but some of it is more curious. One industrial study showed less back pain in workers who attended church regularly (32). A military study showed less back pain in "model soldiers" who had earned 2 or 3 battle stars (17). Some authors feel that there is an increase in the prevalence of back pain among tall individuals (43), whereas others feel that there is a greater chance for developing back pain if the person is short and fat. A review of the data from the larger studies fails to show any significant association at all with body types (18). One hears much about foot problems and back pain, but there are no good data showing a significant relationship (18). One hears much about leg-length discrepancy and back pain, but once again, there are no data to correlate leg-length discrepancy with back pain unless the discrepancy is severe. People have looked at climate as a determinant of back pain. Certain reports show increased incidence of back pain during the spring or autumn (18), whereas in others it occurs during the spring and summer (43). There are additional data to indicate that cold weather and especially wet climates may activate back problems (26). In the final analysis, climate per se does not appear to be a significant determinant for back pain. Psychological factors have been looked at extensively. These are very important and Drs. Toomey and Peterson address them in more detail elsewhere in this volume.

As the list of studies goes on and on and as the data accumulates, it becomes possible to develop a "typical story" of the back pain sufferer. If developed, such a scenario would probably go something like this: The next back pain patient that walks into the office could be anyone from 75% of the population, male or female. The patient's initial episode of pain was probably mild and was resolved without medical attention. He probably developed the first attack of back pain near the end of the third decade, and now that he is approximately 50, many of his friends in his suburban town have a similar story to tell. His occupation is probably not critical, although chances are he is doing heavier rather than lighter work. The patient is more likely to be a truck driver or a nurse than a teacher or salesman. The X-rays might show some disk degeneration at 1 or 2 levels. With treatment he has a 50% chance of getting better within 1 week and a 90% chance of improving within 2 months, regardless of what treatment is rendered. The need for hospitalization would be slight, and the need for surgery at the time of his first visit would be so remote that it need not be mentioned.

CHRONIC BACK PAIN SUFFERER

When one looks at this typical patient, the picture does not look too bad. Although the condition of back pain is ubiquitous, it is self-limited, and it is rare that the patient comes to surgery. However, it must be remembered, as has been previously noted, that although the condition shows a high remission rate, it also shows a high recurrence rate. In addition, although the percentage of people who suffer chronically beyond 6 months is relatively small, the absolute number of patients is huge because the problem is so widespread. Consequently, the impact of the chronic back pain sufferer on the economic and health system is enormous.

In England, more than 2% of the population are estimated to see a general practitioner each year because of back pain (4,10). One out of every 20 visits to a general practitioner's office is for back pain and each new visit results in at least two additional visits (2,31). The number of lost work days in England during a one year period in 1969/1970 totalled over 13,000,000. Male workers lost 75 days per worker per year (5). If industrial surveys are considered, the rate goes up because of the selectivity for heavy work. In Anderson's studies (1,2), the rate of work loss in England's industry is approximately 1½ times the overall national rate.

As might be expected, the rate of work loss from back pain has no less an impact on industry than the rate of hospitalization for back pain has on the health care system. In the United States in 1977, almost 400,000 people were hospitalized in short-stay hospitals with a diagnosis of intervertebral disk displacement (50). This does not include all the patients hospitalized with some other diagnosis that includes the complaint of back pain. This figure alone represents over 1% of all short-stay hospitalizations in that year (50). It is interesting that in the western part of the United States, the rate of hospitalization for disk disease is 50% higher than it is elsewhere in the country (50). As might be expected with this large number of hospitalizations for "disk displacement," the amount of surgery for this condition is also large. In the United States in 1977, 166,000 intervertebral disks were surgically removed (50). This figure does not include cases of spinal fusion or other types of surgery done for disorders of the lumbar spine. In addition, it only includes nonfederal short-stay hospitals and the noninstitutionalized civilian population. Again, in the western part of the country, the rate of disk excision relative to the number of all other operations performed was 50% higher than it was elsewhere in the country. From the figures available, it should be added that disk excision is becoming more common. For instance, in 1973, there were approximately 147,000 intervertebral disks excised, and in 1977, the same statistical survey revealed the 166,000 disk excisions mentioned above (46).

An approximation of the relative frequency of disk excision can be made by comparing its rate with the rate of other commonly performed procedures. In 1975 the number of disks excised was approximately equal to the number of meniscectomies. It was almost half as common as closed reduction without internal fixation of fractures (48).

At this point, recognizing the number of disk excisions performed, one might question how well these patients do following their surgery. Most authors agree that the most important indicator of success following disk excision is the percentage of pain-free patients. Current management is fairly successful in eliminating the sciatic component of the pain. This is not the limiting factor, however, and what appears to be the limiting factor in our success is the persistence of back pain. In this regard, the statistics are disappointing. In 1956, Söderberg (41) published a review of 3,928 previously reported cases. In that study the average percentage of patients achieving pain-free status was 53%. There was a wide range with one optimistic report showing 80% of patients free of pain following surgery. However, if one looks hard and carefully at large numbers of operated patients, a figure of 50% is usually a fairly accurate measure of our success. In a review of 2,500 patients who were treated surgically, Spangford (42) showed that 60% of his patients were pain-free, although at very short follow-up. In Barr's report from the Massachusetts General Hospital (3), only 22% of patients that underwent simple disk excision were free of back pain. Even if he included patients who had "minor complaints," only 64% of patients could be placed in the "essentially free of back symptom" category. Hakelius (14), in a review of patients operated on for herniated lumbar disk at the Karolinska Institute, reported that in a long-term follow-up averaging over 7 years, only 31% of patients were free of back pain. Even if one added to the symptom-free group those patients who were improved but still had mild to moderate symptoms, the "success" rate was still only 52%.

It is not the aim of this report to be especially critical of surgical treatment but simply to be realistic. It is essential to recognize what can be offered to patients under the best of circumstances because when the circumstances are not the best, the results get substantially worse. In a recently published study of a group of Workman's Compensation patients who complained of persistent symptoms following initial surgery, the results with each successive surgery were studied. In this group of patients, beginning with the third operation, most patients were worse following their surgery than prior to it (52).

Thus, despite some optimistic reports to the contrary, it is clear that our treatment for a large number of patients that suffer from chronic and recurrent back pain is not good. There are many for whom the appropriate treatment is uncertain, and for those who require surgery, the success rate is not uniformly good. Consequently, there are a large number of chronic back pain sufferers who experience some type of limitation because of their back ailment. In the United States in 1971, there were approximately 8,000,000 people with some impairment of the back or spine— impairment being defined as a permanent defect or chronic condition causing decrease or loss of ability to perform various functions (45). This represented almost 3.9% of our entire population.

In 1971, Haber (13) published a summary of data gathered in the Social Security Administration Study on causes of disability in the United States. He showed that musculoskeletal conditions are at the top of the list of conditions causing disability between the ages of 18 and 64. Of the musculoskeletal conditions, impairments of the back and spine were a close second to arthritis and rheumatism when all ages were considered. In the younger age group (between 18 and 44 years), impairments of the back and spine were the major cause of morbidity and disability in this country. Even in the older age group (45 to 64 years) back and spine impairments were the third leading cause of disability, still quite significant. In a recently published article on musculoskeletal disorders in the United States, Kelsey et al. (24) reviewed disability allowances that were granted by the Social Security Disability Board in 1973. In this study, it was shown that the condition of "displacement of the intervertebral disk" was the second most common cause of disability award for all people through the age of 49 and the third most common for the group between 50 and 55. It must be recognized here that the category of "displacement of the intervertebral disk" did not include all the remaining causes of back and spine impairments.

In the National Institute of Health Household Survey (47) done nationwide in 1974, impairment of the back and spine was the third leading cause of limitation of activity and severe disability for all ages. Once again, for individuals under 45 years of age, impairment of the back and spine was the leading cause of limitation of activity and severe disability, when all disease categories for both males and females were considered. The problem seems to be on the rise. In the United States, the National Institute of Health Household Survey showed that from the period 1969 through 1976, there was a 50% increase in the prevalence of the condition "displaced intervertebral disk." Over that same period, there was a 20% increase in the incidence of this condition (49). The United States National Safety Council statistics indicate that disabling work injuries are rising at a faster frequency than any other injury. This has become such an epidemic that approximately 2% of all employed individuals have a compensable back injury every year, if recurrences are included (37).

The epidemiological outline presented here has revealed a widespread prevalence of low back pain in industrial societies and has presented an evaluation of the determinants of low back pain and the consequences of this ubiquitous problem. It is this writer's hope that the material discussed in this volume will help us to better understand the pathology and the psychology of this condition and to improve our methods of treatment.

REFERENCES

1. Anderson, J. A. D. (1971): Rheumatism in Industry: a Review. *Br. J. Ind. Med.*, 28:103–121.
2. Anderson, J. A. D. (1976): Back Pain in Industry. *The Lumbar Spine and Back Pain*, edited by M. Jayson, pp. 29–46. Grune & Stratton, New York.
3. Barr, J. S. (1951): Low back and sciatic pain. *J. Bone Joint Surg.*, 33:633–649.
4. Benn, R. T., and Wood, P. H. N. (1972): Statistical Appendix—Digest of Data on the Rheumatic Diseases, 4, Morbidity and Mortality in Hospital Services for Rheumatism Sufferers. *Ann. Rheum. Dis.*, 31:522.
5. Benn, R. T., and Wood, P. H. N. (1975): Pain in the back—an attempt to estimate the size of the problem. *Rheumatol. Rehabil.*, 14:121–128.
6. Dehlin, O., Hedenrud, B., and Horal, J. (1976): Back symptoms in nursing aids in a geriatric hospital. *Scand. J. Rehabil. Med.*, 8:47–53.
7. Dillane, J. B., Fry, J., and Kalton, G. (1966): Acute back syndrome—a study from general practice. *Br. Med. J.*, 3:82–84.
8. Dixon, A. S. J. (1976): Diagnosis of low back pain—sorting the complainers. In: *The Lumbar Spine and Back Pain*, edited by M. Jayson, pp. 77–92. Grune & Stratton, New York.
9. Ferguson, D. (1970): Strain injuries in hospital employees. *Med. J. Aust.*, 1:376–379.
10. Fry, J. (1972): *Back Pain and Soft Tissue Rheumatism*, Advisory Services Colloquium Proceedings. (Advisory Services, Clinical and General, Ltd.), London.
11. Glover, J. R. (1976): Prevention of back pain. *The Lumbar Spine and Back Pain*, edited by M. Jayson, pp. 47–54. Grune & Stratton, New York.
12. Goodsell, J. O. (1967): Correlation of ruptured lumbar disc with occupation. *Clin. Orthop.*, 50:225–229.
13. Haber, L. D. (1971): Disabling effects of chronic disease and impairment. *J. Chronic Dis.*, 24:469–487.
14. Hakelius, A. (1970): Prognosis in sciatics. *Acta Orthop. Scand. (Suppl)*, 129:6–71.
15. Hirsch, C., Jonsson, B., and Lewin, T. (1969): Low-back symptoms in a Swedish female population. *Clin. Orthop.*, 63:171–176.
16. Horal, J. (1969): The clinical appearance of low back disorders in the City of Gothenburg, Sweden. *Acta Orthop. Scand. (Suppl)*, 118:8–73.
17. Hrubec, Z., and Nashold, B. S., Jr. (1975): Epidemiology of lumbar disc lesions in the military in World War II. *Am. J. Epidemiol.*, 102:336–376.
18. Hult, L. (1954): Cervical, dorsal and lumbar spinal syndromes. *Acta Orthop. Scand. (Suppl)*, 17:7–102.
19. Hult, L. (1965): The Munkfors Investigation. *Acta Orthop. Scand. (Suppl)*, 16:1–76.
20. Kelsey, J. L. (1975): An epidemiological study of the relationship between occupation and acute herniated lumbar intervertebral discs. *Int. J. Epidemiol.*, 4:197–205.
21. Kelsey, J. L. (1975): An epidemiological study of acute herniated lumbar intervertebral discs. *Rheumatol. Rehabil.*, 14:144–153.
22. Kelsey, J. L., and Hardy, R. J. (1975): Driving of motor vehicles as a risk factor for acute herniated lumbar intervertebral disc. *Am. J. Epidemiol.*, 102:63–73.
23. Kelsey, J. L., and Ostfield, A. M. (1975): Demographic characteristics of persons with acute herniated lumbar intervertebral disc. *J. Chronic Dis.*, 28:37–50.
24. Kelsey, J. L., White, A. A., Pastides, H., Bisbee, G. E. (1979): The impact of musculoskeletal disorders on the population of the United States. *J. Bone Joint Surg. (Am)*, 61:959–964.

25. Kellgran, J. H., and Lawrence, J. S. (1952): Rheumatism in miners, Part II, *Br. J. Ind. Med.*, 9:197–207.
26. Kellgren, J. H., Lawrence, J. S., and Aiken-Swan, J. (1958): Rheumatic complaints in an urban population. *Ann. Rheum. Dis.*, 17:388–397.
27. Kosiak, M., Aurelous, J. R., and Hartfiel, W. F. (1968): The low back problem. *JOM*, 10:588–593.
28. Lawrence, J. S. (1955): Rheumatism in coal miners. *Br. J. Ind. Med.*, 12:249–261.
29. Lawrence, J. S. (1969): Disc degeneration—its frequency and relationship to symptoms. *Ann. Rheum. Dis.*, 28:121–136.
30. Lawrence, J. S., and Aiken-Swan, J. (1952): Rheumatism in miners, Part I, rheumatic complaints. *Br. J. Ind. Med.*, 9:1–12.
31. Logan, W. P. D., and Cushion, A. A. (1958): Morbidity statistics from general practice, Volume I, *General Register Office Studies on Medical and Population Subjects*, No. 14.
32. Magora, A. (1970): Investigation of the relation between low back pain and occupation. *Indust. Med.*, 39:31–37.
33. Magora, A. (1970): Investigation of the relation between low back pain and occupation. *Indust. Med.*, 39:28–34.
34. Magora, A. (1972): Investigation of the relation between low back pain and occupation, three physical requirements: sitting, standing and weight lifting. *Indust. Med.*, 41:5–9.
35. Magora, A. (1974): Investigation of the relation between low back pain and occupation, six medical histories and symptoms. *Scand. J. Rehabil. Med.*, 6:81–88.
36. Nagi, S. Z., Riley, L. E., and Newby, L. G. (1973): A social epidemiology of back pain in a general population. *J. Chronic Dis.*, 26:769–779.
37. National Safety Council(1976): *Accident Facts*. Chicago, Illinois.
38. Partridge, R. E. H., Anderson, J. A. D., McCarthy, M. A., and Dunthie, J. J. R. (1965): Rheumatism in light industry. *Ann. Rheum. Dis.*, 24:332–340.
39. Rowe, M. L. (1969): Low back pain in industry. *J. Occup. Med.*, 11:161–169.
40. Schmorl, G., and Junghanns, H. (1932): *Die Gesunde und Kranke W. Rebelsäule im Rontgen bild.* Thieme, Leipzing.
41. Söderberg, L., and Sjöberg, S. (1961): On operated herniated lumbar discs. *Acta Orthop. Scand.*, 31:146–152.
42. Spangford, E. V. (1972): The lumbar disc herniation, a computer-aided analysis of 2504 operations. *Acta Ortho. Scand. (Suppl)*, 142:1–95.
43. Tauber, J. (1970): An unorthodox look at backaches. *JOM*, 12:128–130.
44. Troup, J. D. G. (1965): Relation of lumbar spine disorders to heavy manual work and lifting. *Lancet*, 1:857–861.
45. Vital and Health Statistics (1971): Prevalence of selected impairments, United States, 1971. Series 10–Number 99. U.S. Dept. of Health, Education, and Welfare, Washington, D.C.
46. Vital and Health Statistics (1973): Surgical operations in short-stay hospitals, United States, 1973. Series 13-Number 34. U.S. Dept. of Health, Education, and Welfare, Washington, D.C.
47. Vital and Health Statistics (1974): Limitation of activity due to chronic conditions, United States, 1974. Series 10-Number 111. U.S. Dept. of Health, Education, and Welfare, Washington, D.C.
48. Vital and Health Statistics (1975): Surgical operations in short-stay hospitals, United States, 1975. Series 13-Number 34. U.S. Dept. of Health, Education, and Welfare, Washington, D.C.
49. Vital and Health Statistics (1976): Prevalence of chronic skin and musculoskeletal conditions, United States, 1976. Series 10-Number 124. U.S. Dept. of Health, Education and Welfare, Washington, D.C.
50. Vital and Health Statistics (1977): Utilization of short-stay hospitals, Annual Summary of the United States, 1977. Series 13-Number 41. U.S. Dept. of Health, Education, and Welfare, Washington, D.C.
51. W.H.O. (1967): *W.H.O. International Statistical Classification of Diseases*, 2 Volumes, Geneva.
52. Waddell, G., Kummel, E. G., Lotto, W. N., Graham, J. D., Hall, H., and McCulloch, J. A. (1979): Failed lumbar disk surgery following industrial injuries. *J. Bone Joint Surg. (Am)*, 61:201–207.
53. Wood, P. (1976): Epidemiology of low back pain. *The Lumbar Spine and Back Pain*, edited by M. Jayson, pp. 13–28. Grune & Stratton, New York.

Low Back Pain: An Occupational Perspective

James L. Schaepe

The Norton Company, Worcester, Massachusetts 01606

There is a consensus among occupational physicians that low back pain syndrome is one of the most burdensome, frequent, and problem-filled entities seen at the workplace. The extent of this problem is enormous. At the outset, it should be mentioned that by the age of 65 at least 50% of workers will be affected by low back pain. Low back pain seems to occur at about the same frequency at work and away from the workplace. It is the leading cause of chronic disability between the ages of 19 and 45 years. In fact, low back pain is the most common complaint treated by family physicians in the United States and is the eleventh ranked cause of hospitalization. The economic dimensions of low back pain syndrome (LBPS) are immense. Approximately $14,000,000,000 was spent on the treatment of low back pain syndrome in the United States in 1978.

It is difficult to obtain statistics regarding LBPS in the United States. However, according to the National Safety Council, approximately 400,000 of 590,000 cases of trunk injury resulted in LBPS in 1979 (1). Approximately 30% of all compensation claims are paid on LBPS claims. Compensation rates for LBPS in Wisconsin rose from 8% of the total cases in 1938 to 19% in 1965 and to 28% in 1978. According to the Eastman Kodak Company of Rochester, New York, LBPS is second only to the common respiratory infection as a source of lost time payment claims. The injury rate yielding LBPS in light industry is approximately 3 to 5 injuries per 1,000 workers per year. In heavy industry, there are up to 200 low back injuries per 1,000 workers per year. In the Norton Company, which is representative of heavy industry, over 100 cases of LBPS are seen each year out of an employee population of approximately 5,000. The estimated direct and indirect costs of LBPS in this company amounts to $250,000 per year. With some 24,000 workers worldwide, the company spends close to $1,000,000 yearly because of the condition.

What is the reason for this increase of LBPS in a society that supposedly has the advantages of automation? One probably has to look at the effects of automation itself to find the answer. A look at technology will confirm that it is a two-edged sword. On one hand, assembly lines are poorly designed, with inadequate safety devices, whereas, on the other hand, technology allows people to be much less physically active in general. It has been said that only 5% of the American population engages in enough physical activity to be called physically fit. Technology is one of the keys to the problem. What is needed is more technology at the worksite and less dependency on it outside.

Traditionally, industry has approached the problem of low back pain by focusing on the worker. His medical history, physical exam, and back X-rays are used as screening tools for employment. Once the person is hired, he or she may be trained or educated how to lift properly. However, in 1978, Snook, an ergonomist, published a study showing that traditional industrial methods, i.e., selection and education, are really of no value in reducing the incidence of LBPS (9). The ergonomist is a person who brings a multidisciplinary approach from the sciences of biomedical engineering, physiology, psychology, and anatomy to bear upon the relationship between job and worker. The ergonomic approach is to fit the job to the worker and not vice versa. In his study, Snook demonstrated a 30% reduction in low back injuries when jobs were selected so that 75% of the work force could do a job without undue effort. Through laboratory studies for which he engaged hundreds of subjects to lift tote boxes of known weight, he developed psychophysical lift tables. These enabled him to gauge the amount that a worker can lift without his perception of undue effort. Snook's tables are being used increasingly throughout industry.

The ergonomic approach emphasizes the workplace and the worker. Both aspects are equally important. I believe that the traditional methods of evaluating people—using a history, an examination, and X-rays—are of limited value. There are particular risk factors that give rise to the LBPS. There is also a summation of risk factors that, if reduced, leads to a predictable decrease in the incidence of the syndrome.

Dr. Brooks, Professor of Technology of Social Institutions at Harvard, notes that technology offers a society options, and a strong value system operating within a

(RISK FACTORS AFFECTING LOAD)

I. Physical work environment

   A. Task load

   B. Immediate work area

PLUS

II. Psychosocial work environment

PLUS

(RISK FACTORS AFFECTING CAPACITY)

III. Personal risk factors

FIG. 1.

society can select those options (2). Technology can be disastrous in a society where a weak value system exists together with a relative lack of concern for the worker (2). The value system present at the worksite dictates the level of care provided there. It is the duty of the occupational physician to help bring to the work environment those values that allow new knowledge to be readily utilized. Concern for quality of work life has to be the prime consideration at the workplace; improved quantity of output will then naturally follow.

An understanding of the physical work environment, psychosocial work environment, and the susceptibilities of the individual worker were used to develop a set of risk factors leading to LBPS (Fig. 1).

PHYSICAL WORK ENVIRONMENT RISK FACTORS

Weight To Be Lifted

The amount of weight to be lifted is a very important factor (Fig. 2). For example, lifting more than 45 lb doubles the chance that a low back injury will occur. According to Snook's psychophysical lift tables (9), 75% of male workers can lift 45 lb and push a horizontal weight of 69 lb without undue effort; the statistics for women are 33 lb and 52 lb, respectively. This information was used in 1978 during a discussion with the Norton Company's Manager of Health and Safety and other safety personnel; the result was a directive stating that no worker should lift weights greater than 35 lb. This directive was ludicrous, because a visit to a worksite where many back injuries originated revealed people who were routinely pushing or rolling 350-lb barrels of material.

PHYSICAL WORK ENVIRONMENT

1. Exact weight to be lifted

2. Height of lift

3. Distance from body of lift

4. Speed of lift

5. Frequency of lift

6. Symmetry of lift

7. Job requirement postures

8. Micro environment
   Temperature
   Floor surface

FIG. 2.

The issue here is: What is the value system operating at the workplace? Our system has to be humane as well as efficient. If a given work organization values the quality of work life, changes such as limitations on lifting will evolve. If not, then society will ultimately enact laws to achieve that effect. In 1976, the Work Environment Law was passed in Norway, specifying what should and should not be done at the worksite.

Height of Lift

About 66% of lifting, according to Snook's study (9), is below knuckle height, i.e., below approximately 31 inches, and 70% of the back injuries at the worksite are caused by these low lifts. Thus, low lifts are an important factor.

Distance of Body From Lift

Snook's study also indicates that the pressure generated upon the intravertebral disk is 33% greater when the arms are outstretched than when the object is lifted from the floor but kept close to the body. Thus, the lifting distance from the body's center of gravity is an important risk factor. Workers are often taught correct lifting techniques, but this training is useless if, in fact, the work conditions do not allow them to bring the weight to be lifted close to the body.

Speed of Lift

When something is lifted rapidly, there is up to a 15 to 20% increase in the actual weight being lifted (4). Workers should be advised to lift heavy objects in a slow and deliberate manner.

Frequency of Lift

Frequency of lift relates to metabolic output and is also a risk factor. The more frequently a task is undertaken within a time period, the less efficient the worker becomes. One study showed that people doing even light work, such as operating a light drill press, showed decreased efficiency as the week progressed; by Friday they had lost 10 to 15% of their efficiency. Therefore, if one adjusts work schedules to the ability pattern of the worker, there will be fewer low back injuries. Another study, discussed in Zenz's *Textbook of Occupational Medicine*, was undertaken at the new Russian Fiat assembly line plant (10). Workers were found to be least efficient in their first hour of work, after which time they remained on an efficient plateau until lunch break. After lunch, there was another period of 20 min before workers again reached top capacity, and this was maintained until the last half hour of work, when efficiency again dropped. These findings were used to adjust the speed of the assembly line to reflect the efficiency pattern of the assembly line workers.

Symmetry of Lift

Donald Chaffin at the Engineering Human Performance Laboratory at the University of Michigan has pointed out that although there are no conclusive studies, evidence indicates that an asymmetrical lift causes more back injury than a symmetrical lift, i.e., a lift centered in front of a person (4). Perhaps this seems obvious, but it is information upon which we could improve with additional research.

Job Posture

Any job that requires a fixed position—whether sitting, standing, or bending—leads to an increased number of back injuries. Leaning forward so as to decrease the body height by 20% increases the energy output by 30 to 50%. This leads to fatigue and increased injuries (10).

The Trunk Twist

There are jobs that require a twisting turn of the body; in these, if the worker is in a hurry to execute the maneuver, there will be a moment at which stress on the back is markedly increased. Some machines, such as presses, are constructed to prevent the worker from standing too close, which, of course, is counter to one of the main rules in lifting, namely, to bring the object as close as possible to the body. Another rule is, whenever possible, to lift the object between the legs, so that there is no distance from the object to the center of gravity of the body. When placing the object between the legs is not possible, it is equally effective to use the classical "bend your knees and keep your back straight" way of lifting. There is no more adverse pressure on the back with this last method of lifting than there is with the method of bending and lifting the item close to the body. However, in many instances, there is no way that the worker can bring things close to him while lifting. Some workers are lifting as much as 100 lb with each lift and doing so with improper technique because of the design of the machinery or process.

Immediate Environment

When the temperature is increased, metabolic output is increased. This increased output leads to muscle fatigue that, in turn, leads to decreased muscular coordination and increased injury. Noise is another problem. Work noises can be irritating, leading to muscular tension and fatigue as well as to emotional stress. These causes of environmental stress can decrease the worker's reserves making him or her more vulnerable to injury of any sort, including LBPS.

While walking through a plant recently, I noticed a man rolling a 350-lb barrel filled with abrasive material. Rolling these barrels is his job for the entire day. This barrel rolling is an example of underutilization of available technology. Previously sharp-edged barrels were used, but those were replaced by barrels with rounded edges, making them easier to roll. This may be classified as quarterway technology—it has not reached the halfway mark. In another area of the plant, two men were lifting a 160-lb vat. There is a safety device that is intended for use when the vat is to be lifted; however, using the safety device requires more time and it is therefore usually bypassed. Such safety devices represent halfway technology; they are designed "after the fact" and are added on to a particular process, thereby slowing it down, making it cumbersome and inefficient for workers to use. An increase in the incorporation of bioengineering into the workings of the worksite will go far to obviate poorly designed, unsafe machines and processes.

Because of the increasing number of women in industry, it is the aim of the Office of Equal Opportunity to have women working in all areas of the workplace. However, at present, there are jobs in our plants that only 4 to 5% of women can do. Selection of appropriate men and women for those jobs is a pressing problem. The medical department in our company is attempting to introduce strength testing as the most appropriate available technology. However, some people feel that strength testing is discriminatory. Strength testing will be cautiously used by industry until its acceptance can be assured by a resolution of the diverse viewpoints of such government agencies as the Office of Equal Opportunity and the National Institute of Occupational Safety and Health (for a discussion of strength testing, see W. M. Keyserling, *this volume*).

PSYCHOSOCIAL WORK ENVIRONMENT RISK FACTORS

The psychosocial work environment is derived from the work organization and structure (Fig. 3). Job security is the primary concern of the worker. Next to job security comes fear of injury and poor health (9). Monotony is also a concern as is the lack of control or input into one's job situation. If one is overcontrolled by a job and cannot leave for a few minutes without falling behind in the work, the results can be very stressful. Overcontrol by a supervisor to the point where one cannot take time away from a job is similarly stressful. When there is psychological work stress, LBPS is twice as frequent (7). Individuals who feel alienated from their work and who do not find enjoyment in their job content are stressed, and they have twice the incidence of LBPS. Stress leads to nervous tension and simultaneously to increased muscle tension. In addition, there is an over-recruitment of muscles that are not actually needed for the job but that are called into play in

PSYCHOSOCIAL WORK ENVIRONMENT

1. Degree of job security

2. Degree of work stimulation

3. Degree of freedom of movement

4. Degree of input of abilities and education

FIG. 3.

such circumstances. This overuse of muscles, typical of tense people, leads to increased muscle fatigue and a higher incidence of LBPS. Stress-induced fatigue is also responsible for a decreased quality of life away from work. People are less apt to be socially or politically active or to have creative hobbies, particularly if they feel alienated from work and carry home a higher level of anxiety and fatigue.

INDIVIDUAL RISK FACTORS

A relationship between personal attitudes and incidence of LBPS has been implicated. According to Kobasa et al (6), people who are in touch with their feelings, who feel they have input into the direction of their lives, and who are not threatened by change are shown to have a third as much illness following highly stressful situations. A study by House and Wells (5) showed that in those individuals who have at least one other person functioning as a support system, there was little or no physical illness following periods of high psychosocial stress, despite the amount of stress present at work (Fig. 4). However, generally, stress has been shown to lead to increased illness and accidents. Stress certainly comes from the work environment, but how the person responds to it is a key factor in the resulting incidence of illness, accidents, and LBPS.

Psychological and sociological factors influence the person's behavioral characteristics. Those individuals who have a confidant are more likely to discuss their stresses with that person. Their patterns of nutrition and physical fitness are also likely to be improved by a positive social support situation. In short, they are better able to cope.

In a study of physical fitness in a group of Los Angeles County fire fighters, Cady et al (3) found that over a 3-yr period only 10% of back injuries occurred in those who were most physically fit, compared with those who were least physically fit (Fig. 5. Evidently, muscular strength is protective. However, muscular strength is reduced to approximately half of peak strength by age 55 years. Thus, the age

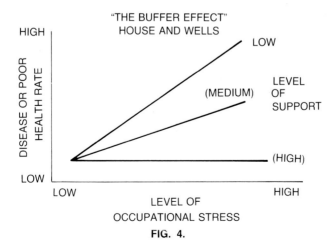

FIG. 4.

SUBSEQUENT TO EXAMINATION

	Most Fit	Middle Fit	Least Fit
No. injured	2	36	19
Percent	.77	3.19	7.14
Cost	$147,400	$178,993	$106,821
Cost per injury	$73,700	$ 4,972	$ 5,622
Total	266	1127	259

FIG. 5.

of the worker is a significant factor in deciding what a person can safely lift. The individual risk factors are listed in Fig. 6.

The following conclusions can be drawn regarding reducing the incidence of LBPS at the worksite. First, an equal emphasis has to be placed on identifying and reducing environmental and individual-related risk factors that are operative at the worksite. Second, a worksite value system that places high priority on quality of work life will insure that the necessary amount of effort is spent on improving the work environment and encouraging the worker to adopt a healthier lifestyle.

This discussion has been a preliminary attempt to define the causes of LBPS in terms of relatively simple risk factors. More research is required to validate these observations.

INDIVIDUAL RISK FACTORS

1. Psychological -- attitude
2. Behavioral -- coping patterns
3. Postural -- lordosis
4. Physical fitness
5. Muscular strength
6. Age

FIG. 6.

REFERENCES

1. *Accidental Facts* (1979): National Safety Council, Chicago, Illinois, pp. 4–24.
2. Brooks, H. (1980): Modern technology: Problems or opportunity? *Daedalus*, 109:41–82.
3. Cady, L., Bischoff, D. P., O'Connell, E. R., Thomas, P. C. (1979): Strength and physical fitness and subsequent back injuries in fire fighters. *JOM*, 21:269–272.
4. Chaffin, D. (1977): Degenerative disease and injury to the back. In: *Occupational Health and Safety Symposium*. D.H.E.W. (NIOSH) Pub. No. 78-169, p. 54.

5. House, J., and Wells, J. (1977): Occupational stress, social support, and health. In: *Reducing Occupational Stress*. D.H.E.W. (NIOSH) Pub. No. 78-140.
6. Kobasa, S. C., Hilker, R. J., and Maddi, S. R. (1977): Job stress and work performance. In: *Occupational Health and Safety Symposium*. D.H.E.W. (NIOSH) Pub. No. 78-169, pp. 114–122.
7. Nerell, G., and Waghlund, I. (1979): Stress factors in the working environments of white collar workers. In: *Reducing Occupational Stress*. D.H.E.W. (NIOSH) Pub. No. 78-140, pp. 62–72.
8. Shostok, A. (1978): Blue collar stressors, workplace stress, reforms and prospects. In: *Reducing Occupational Stress*. D.H.E.W. (NIOSH) Pub. No. 78-140, pp. 73–85.
9. Snook, S., Campbell, R. A., and Hart, J. W. (1978): A study of three preventative approaches to low back injury. *JOM*, 20:478–481.
10. Zenz, Carl (1975): *Occupational Medicine, Principles and Practical Applications*, p. 538. Yearbook Medical Publishers, Chicago, Illinois.

Chronic Low Back Pain, edited by
M. Stanton-Hicks and Robert Boas.
Raven Press, New York © 1982.

Five-Year Follow-Up Status of Chronic Low Back Pain Patients

*Timothy C. Toomey, **Ann Gill Taylor, †J. A. Skelton,
and *Harold Carron

*Department of Anesthesiology, School of Medicine, and **School of Nursing,
University of Virginia, Charlottesville, Virginia 22908; and †Department of Psychology,
Dickinson College, Carlisle, Pennsylvania 17013

Long-term follow-up studies of the physical and psychosocial adjustment of the patient treated for chronic pain are rarely reported in the literature. A few studies have reported improvement in psychological (14) and physical function (3,11,12) in patients following pain clinic treatment programs. However, in no case is the follow-up period greater than 3 years, and the majority of reports are based on in-patient treatment models. No study has reported a long-term comparison of results over two time periods following an out-patient model of treatment.

The current report is an extension of an earlier, 2-year follow-up study of patients with low back pain treated with nerve blocks in the pain clinic setting (1). This earlier study reported generally positive therapeutic outcomes following nerve-block treatment, especially in view of the chronicity and intractability of the patients treated. The study also noted extensive gender-associated differences in treatment outcomes, with women reporting generally more positive outcomes than men. The initial study emphasized the need for employing multiple criteria of functioning in assessing the effectiveness of nerve-block therapy.

This review extends the period of follow-up from the original survey by 3 years. By measuring a variety of functional determinants, this 5-year study investigated whether the chronic pain state improves, stabilizes, or deteriorates as a consequence of time elapsed after treatment. It also tried to determine if sex-related differences in outcome maintain themselves over time. Another important purpose was to ascertain the criteria that patients associated with improvement or nonimprovement over an extended period of time. A final intent was to determine the association between behavioral reports of improved functioning versus the more global ratings of overall change in pain intensity and frequency often employed as the only outcome criteria in many studies reported in the literature.

Dr. Toomey's present address: Pain Clinic, Dental Research Unit, Bldg. 210H, University of North Carolina, Chapel Hill, North Carolina 27514.

The present report is not a controlled study of nerve-block efficacy in patients with low back pain. Indeed, a number of such studies have been reported (2,4,8,16). As emphasized in the previous follow-up with this patient sample (5), the focus of the present research is on multiple indices of treatment effectiveness, in addition to pain reduction. Although responses obtained in the present study cannot be ascribed to nerve-block treatments administered 5 years earlier, the data do permit a look at the extended course of the chronic pain state in individuals presenting themselves at an earlier time to a pain treatment center. Such data are of considerable normative interest and can be employed in broadly based comparisons with other centers, which utilize different therapeutic models or patient populations.

METHOD

Respondents

The pool of respondents in the present study is described in detail in the original follow-up (1). That study presented 2-year follow-up data on 151 individuals who were treated with epidural or subarachnoid nerve block for low back pain not caused by malignancy. The initial follow-up contact occurred in 1974. In 1978, the same group of patients was contacted by mail and was requested to complete a second questionnaire. Approximately 45% ($N = 70$) of 1974 respondents also returned the 1978 questionnaire, which is somewhat lower than the 65% response rate to the original survey.

In view of the potential for self-selection biases in the present sample, an analysis of the 1974 questionnaires was performed to determine if the 1978 respondents and nonrespondents differed in any systematic way during the initial follow-up study. These data are presented in the results section.

Although 70 individuals returned the 1978 follow-up questionnaire, the number replying to any particular questionnaire item ranged from as few as 9 to as many as 66. Both the variation in effective sample size and the self-selected nature of the respondent sample seriously compromise statistical assumptions concerning random sampling. Therefore, statistical interpretation of data obtained in the present study has been kept to a minimum.

Questionnaire

The present questionnaire was designed to be comparable with the earlier instrument. It included self-ratings—typically in a Likert-type format—of pain frequency and intensity and self-evaluations of functional status, e.g., ability to walk, to bend, to work, and to engage in social and recreational activities. Respondents were asked to indicate their involvement in litigation related to their back pain, but too few responses to this series were obtained to make analysis worthwhile. Respondents were also asked to indicate the amount of medication used for pain relief, the number of medications used for pain relief, the number of additional operations undertaken since nerve-block treatment, and other treatment sought for pain relief.

Plan of Analysis

A strength of the present study is that follow-up data for the respondent sample are available for the years 1974 and 1978. In order to assess the stability versus change over time in replies to questionnaire items, most of the analyses that follow examine replies as a function of time. In addition to the concern with change in respondent ratings over time, the present study also sought to examine sex differences in responses to questionnaire items. Since there were clear tendencies toward differential responding by males and females to many of the items on the 1974 questionnaire, the analyses of the present study are also reported with regard to the sex of the respondents.

RESULTS

1978 Respondents versus Nonrespondents

A stepwise discriminant analysis was performed to determine if consistent differences existed between individuals who replied only to the 1974 follow-up questionnaire and those who replied to both the 1974 and 1978 surveys. Of 32 potential predictor variables obtained from the 1974 questionnaire, three were significant in predicting 1978 respondent versus nonrespondent status. These included respondents' ages, ratings of posttreatment improvement in ability to bend, and estimates of the amount of medication taken. These data are presented in Table 1.

The data indicate that the 1978 respondent group does not fully represent the larger 1974 follow-up group but that it is similar to the larger group on over 90% of the 1974 questionnaire items. With respect to sample composition by sex, the present survey's composition of 67% females is comparable with the original follow-up group, which was 61% female.

TABLE 1. *Means for discriminating variables: 1978 respondents vs. nonrespondents*

	Respondent status in 1978[a]	
Variable	Respondents	Nonrespondents
Age in 1974	50.5	45.7
	(11.2)[b]	(12.3)
Ability to bend[c]	2.9	2.3
	(1.3)	(1.4)
Amount of medication in 1974[d]	1.3	1.0
	(1.1)	(1.1)

[a]N respondents = 70; N nonrespondents = 77.
[b]Standard deviations shown in parentheses.
[c]Higher means indicate improved functioning.
[d]Lower means indicate less medication.

Frequency and Intensity of Pain

Ratings of pain frequency were made on a 6-point Likert scale, where $1 =$ no pain and $6 =$ constant pain. Respondents' ratings were combined into three frequency ratings: before treatment (retrospectively), at the original follow-up, and on 5-year follow-up (Fig. 1).

The three ratings were analyzed via a multivariate profile analysis, with sex of respondent as the independent variable. Results indicate that males and females did not differ in overall frequency ratings ($F < 1$) nor in the degree to which adjacent ratings changed (multivariate $F < 1$). However, pretreatment ratings differed significantly from 1974 posttreatment ratings (F (1,62) $= 38.68$, $p < .001$). There was no significant change in frequency ratings between 1974 and the 5-year follow-up. It may be concluded that perceived pain frequency declines in the initial period following treatment and remains stable over time.

Pain intensity was rated at three levels: (a) pain as usually experienced, (b) pain at its worst, and (c) pain at its least. A 6-point Likert scale was used; the scale anchors were "no pain" and "unbearable pain." Respondents' ratings of "usual" pain were combined into three intensity groupings of mild, moderate, and severe. Figure 2 presents the intensity ratings across the three periods surveyed.

A profile analysis indicated no significant differences in the intensity ratings of males and females. However, pretreatment ratings differed significantly from 1974 posttreatment ($F(1,37) = 56.59$, $p < .001$). There was no significant change in intensity ratings between 1974 and the 5-year follow-up. Similar to frequency ratings, pain intensity declined in the initial period after treatment and remained stable over time. It is interesting that both males and females were equally likely to employ the extreme end of the frequency dimension to describe their pain prior to treatment, but only females tended to employ the more extreme end of the intensity dimension to describe pain experienced before treatment. Furthermore, the 5-year

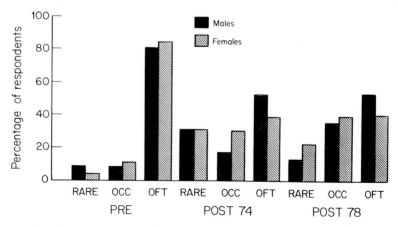

FIG. 1. Percentage of respondents indicating rare, occasional, or frequent episodes of pain pretreatment (PRE), posttreatment 1974 (POST 74), and posttreatment 1978 (POST 78), *N* Males = 22 (PRE), 23(74), 22(78); *N* Females = 44 (PRE), 46(74), 44(78).

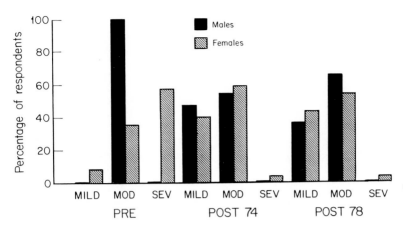

FIG. 2. Percentage of respondents indicating mild, moderate, or severe intensity of pain pretreatment (PRE), posttreatment 1974 (POST 74), and posttreatment 1978 (POST 78). *N* Males = 14 (PRE), 13(74), 14(78); *N* Females = 35 (PRE), 33(74), 30(78).

follow-up indicated a continuation of the trend in the original study for ratings of pain intensity to decrease more than ratings of pain frequency.

Functional-Behavioral Improvements

A number of authors have emphasized the need for functional-behavioral measures in evaluating the rehabilitation of chronic pain patients (6,7,12,15). The present survey assessed respondents' current functioning in four classes of behavior deemed relevant to their pain state. These included measures of physical abilities (down-time, ability to bend, ability to walk), vocational abilities (time lost from work), avocational ability (recreational and social activity), and health-seeking behaviors (number of surgeries and medication usage). With the exception of the last category, respondents were asked to employ a 5-point scale for each behavior assessed. The scale anchors were "function completely improved or restored" and "function worse than before treatment." In view of the relatively small sample size, responses were grouped into two classes, improved or unimproved. Responses indicating no change or deterioration in function were classed as unimproved and other responses were classed as improved.

Physical Abilities

Down-Time

Of the present sample, 56 members (80%) reported in 1974 that prior to nerve-block treatment they had spent some days in bed because of pain. Prior to treatment, males and females did not differ appreciably on this measure. Of the 52 individuals who replied to both the 1974 and 1978 posttreatment down-time items, 32 (62%) classified themselves as improved on both surveys. Eight persons classifying them-

FIVE-YEAR FOLLOW-UP

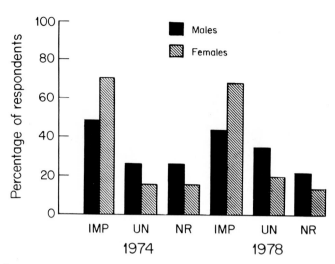

FIG. 3. Percentage of respondents indicating improvement (IMP), unimprovement (UN), and no response (NR) in down-time in 1974 and 1978. *N* Males = 17 (1974), 18 (1978); *N* Females = 40 (1974), 41 (1978).

selves as improved in 1974 changed to unimproved in 1978 (15%). Five individuals (10%) changed from the unimproved to improved category over this period. Although not statistically significant, there was a trend for males in both posttreatment surveys to indicate less improvement in down-time. The data are reported in Fig. 3.

Ability to Bend and Walk

For both of these important abilities, the initial follow-up trend showing that over half of the sampled females reported improvement was also observed in the 5-year follow-up survey. The ability to bend continued in 1978 to be the behavior on which both sexes reported lowest improvement ratings, with 39% of the males and 62% of the females reporting improvement in both surveys. Ability to walk is the only item on which a statistically significant sex difference emerged in both surveys. The 44% improvement rate noted among males in the 1974 survey declined to 35% in 1978. Females reported a 68% and a 66% improvement rate in 1974 and 1978, respectively. It appears that males either have more severe physical impairment associated with their back pain or are more conservative in reporting physical gains than females. Figures 4 and 5 allow ready comparison of the data for males and females.

Vocational Ability

Both males and females reported gains in this category of functioning on the 5-year follow-up study (Fig. 6). Most striking is the substantial increase from 1974

FIVE-YEAR FOLLOW-UP

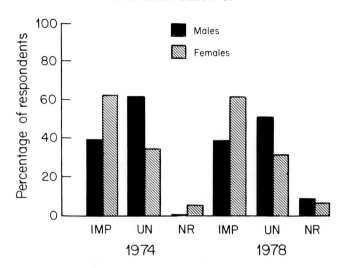

FIG. 4. Percentage of respondents indicating improvement (IMP), unimprovement (UN), and no response (NR) in ability to bend in 1974 and 1978. *N Males = 23 (1974), 21 (1978); N Females = 45 (1974), 44 (1978).*

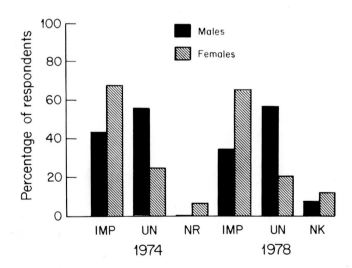

FIG. 5. Percentage of respondents indicating improvement (IMP), unimprovement (UN), and no response (NR) in ability to walk in 1974 and 1978. *N Males = 23 (1974), 21 (1978); N Females = 44 (1974), 41 (1978).*

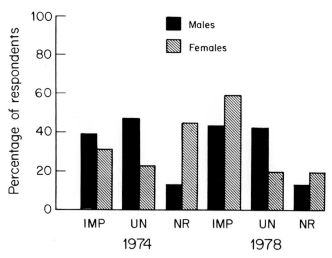

FIG. 6. Percentage of respondents indicating improvement (IMP), unimprovement (UN), and no response (NR) in time lost from work in 1974 and 1978. *N* Males = 20 (1974), 20 (1978); *N* Females = 26 (1974), 38 (1978).

to 1978 in the percentage of females classifying themselves as improved in their ability to work (32% vs 62%). This is concomitant with a decline in the percentage of females failing to reply to an item assessing amount of time lost from work over the survey periods (45% in 1974 vs 19% in 1978). The results suggest that as many as 11 women enjoyed increased ability to work in the 1974 to 1978 period. This may be partially associated with the increased general trend for females to join the work force. However, the item relates work ability to pain relief and does not specify nature of work. Males, conversely, showed only marginal improvement in this ability, with 39% improvement in 1974 and 44% in 1978.

Avocational Abilities

Recreational and social abilities may be viewed, in relative terms, as the least essential functions assessed in the present survey. Males continued to report substantially less improvement on these items. In the 1974 survey, a statistically significant sex difference emerged between male and female improvement in recreational ability (30% vs 55%). In the 5-year follow-up, the sex difference was marginally significant, with 39% of the males reporting improvement compared with 51% improvement in females. This is consistent with males' response conservatism on the more physically essential abilities such as walking. Both males and females reported somewhat greater improvement in social activity ability. Improvement rates for males were 39% in 1974 and 48% in 1978, whereas among females they were 64% and 70% for the two time periods (Figs. 7 and 8).

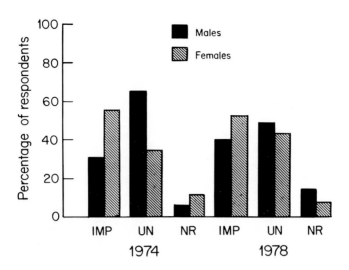

FIG. 7. Percentage of respondents indicating improvement (IMP), unimprovement (UN), and no reply (NR), in recreational ability in 1974 and 1978. *N* Males = 22 (1974), 20 (1978); *N* Females = 42 (1974), 44 (1978).

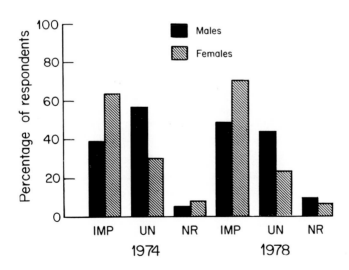

FIG. 8. Percentage of respondents indicating improvement (IMP), unimprovement (UN), and no reply (NR) in social activity ability in 1974 and 1978. *N* Males = 22 (1974), 21 (1978); *N* Females = 44 (1974), 44 (1978).

Health-Seeking Behaviors

Respondents were asked in 1974 and 1978 to indicate the number of additional operations for low back pain. They were also asked to indicate the amount of medication taken for back pain. Although some 23 of the original 151 patients on the 1974 survey reported one or more surgical procedures for pain, on the 5-year survey only three respondents reported additional operations. This change represented a substantial reduction over time in this aspect of chronic pain behavior. The reduction in the number of surgical procedures may be viewed as a generally encouraging finding, since approximately 21% of patients reporting surgery *prior* to nerve-block treatment noted that they were *worse* following nerve block.

A total of 45 patients responded to the medication usage items in the 1974 and 1978 surveys. Five-year follow-up revealed increasing stability in the pattern of medication usage over time, with 24 (53%) of the patients reporting that they used the same amount in 1978 as in 1974. In the original survey, 38% reported taking the same amount as before treatment. Eleven patients (24%) reported taking less medication in 1978 than 1974. Ten patients (23%) reported taking more medication in 1978 than 1974. The first follow-up noted that 29% of the sample reported taking more medication in 1974 than before treatment. Thus, medication usage appears to be a somewhat characteristic feature of chronic pain patients over an extended period of time. No reliable sex differences emerged on this variable in the present survey.

Overall Improvement

1978 respondents were classified into two groups based on their replies to a 5-point scale item asking for a rating of overall improvement in their chronic pain condition. Those indicating no improvement or worsening of pain were classed as unimproved ($N = 19$), whereas the remaining respondents were classed as improved ($N = 46$). A stepwise discriminant analysis was performed on a pool of demographic, pain rating, and functional-behavioral variables to determine the criteria associated with ratings of improvement and nonimprovement. A series of six discriminating variables emerged and the resultant model correctly classified over 90% of respondents into the appropriate improvement category. Table 2 presents the variables and their partial correlations (r's) with improvement status.

Table 2 indicates that the best variables for predicting self-perceived improvement are (a) change in rated frequency of pain from 1974 pretreatment to 1974 post-treatment (frequency change) and (b) change from 1974 to 1978 in estimated amount of time spent in bed due to pain (down-time change). For both variables, the greater the positive change, the greater the likelihood of respondents to rate themselves as improved. The two variables are capable of correctly classifying 87.7% of respondents into the appropriate improvement category.

The four remaining variables in Table 2 also contributed significantly to the discrimination of improved from unimproved respondents. Thus, females were more likely to rate themselves as improved than were males (sex). The more improvement

TABLE 2. *Variables discriminating improved from unimproved respondents*

Variable[a]	Partial r[b]	Multiple R[c]
Frequency change	.48	.48
Down-time change	.57	.69
Sex	.33	.73
Work change	.32	.77
Staff sympathy	− .25	.78
Worst change	− .26	.80

[a]Variables listed in the order of their inclusion in the discriminant equation.
[b]An index of the unique contribution of a variable to the discriminant equation, after controlling for the effects of variables already in the equation.
[c]An index of the incremental strength of each variable in the discriminant equation.

a respondent noted from 1974 to 1978 in ability to work (work change), the more likely he or she was to be a member of the improved category. Interestingly, the more sympathetic and understanding a respondent viewed pain clinic staff to be (staff sympathy), the *less* likely the respondent was to be a member of the improved category. Finally, the greater the decrease from pretreatment to posttreatment rating of pain intensity "at its worst" (worst change), the more likely a respondent was to be improved. Adding the four additional variables to the prediction equation increased the percentage of correctly classified respondents to 92.3%.

The above variables are generally consistent with common sense criteria that patients might employ in determining improvement status. It is of interest that both a global pain rating variable (perceived frequency change) and a functional variable (change in down-time) emerged as the most powerful predictors. Sex and work change as predictor variables are consistent with data presented earlier. The meaning of the perceived sympathy variable is not at all obvious and could probably not be explained without resorting to considerable *post hoc* speculation. Such a finding, however, is intriguing and suggests a direction for further study of chronic pain patients with methodologies developed by other investigators to assess perceived "metness" of needs in the physician-patient dyad (10).

DISCUSSION

The present data indicate generally favorable long-term results among patients presenting themselves for nerve-block treatment in an integrated pain clinic setting. Subjective ratings indicating improvement, a low percentage of surgical intervention, and enhanced ability to work in over half the sample attest to the positive outcomes of treatment. The temporal framework within which perceived improvements occurred emphasizes the importance of long-term follow-up studies. Subjective ratings of pain frequency and intensity showed the greatest improvement immediately following nerve-block treatment, as evidenced by the emergence of the variables frequency change and worst change as significant discriminators of improved versus unimproved respondents. Functional improvement, on the other hand, occurred more slowly, perhaps as a result of patients' gradually "trying out" functions that had been previously limited by their pain state. Thus, improvements in down-time and work-related abilities occurring between the initial and the present follow-up also discriminated improved from unimproved respondents.

Gender-associated differences in functional ability continued to be noted in the present survey, with females generally reporting enhanced improvement status in comparison with males. Males appear to be particularly conservative in reporting improvement on the most and least essential functions assessed, i.e., ability to walk and recreational ability. Nevertheless, the percentage of males who classified themselves as improved increased for most functions across the two surveys, and the number of functional abilities demonstrating a significant sex difference declined as well. This suggests that males are decidedly more conservative than females in reporting improvement on a wide spectrum of abilities but that some conservatism tends to wane over time.

As noted in the original follow-up (1), the reasons for such gender differences are unclear. It is possible that the pain states of males are associated with greater levels of physical impairment. Some support for this may be adduced from the finding in the original follow-up that onset of pain for the majority of males was associated with work-related accidents, a setting predictably associated with potential for severe back injury. As noted by several authors (5,9,13,17), the role of litigation is a complex variable affecting treatment outcome in chronic pain patients, and work-related injuries among male respondents would likely be associated with this factor. A final point concerns the differential meaning of chronic pain and disability for males and females. Males with chronic pain may have a greater need to maintain attitudes and behaviors consistent with more profound levels of impairment to offset the cultural stereotype requiring males to be more physically robust and vocationally productive than females. The fact that the majority of the respondents in the sample came from conservative, working-class backgrounds and that their pain conditions frequently interfered with traditional male roles, e.g., ability to work, lends credence to this hypothesis.

Results from the 5-year follow-up corroborate the observation made during the initial follow-up that the isolated criteria of pain reduction and/or return to work are too narrow for assessment of patient outcome. The present data revealed rather wide variation among subjective and behavioral ratings of improvement as a consequence of the particular function being assessed. Results of the discriminant analysis assessing variables associated with improvement and nonimprovement revealed the complexity of factors associated with response to treatment. Both the pain reduction variable of rated pain frequency and the behavioral variable of time spent in bed were of equal importance in predicting treatment outcome. This also suggests that patients are inclined to judge improvement in terms of reduced exposure time to pain and enhanced physical functioning, leading support to behaviorally based treatment programs (6,7) that emphasize increased levels of physical activity and inattention to pain-related behaviors. As noted earlier, results of the discriminant analysis suggests that the complex variable of patient perception of the physician is also related to improvement status and future studies should be undertaken to explore the association of this dimension to treatment outcome.

The data presented in this report are best understood as an extended view of the patient with chronic pain who, at a considerably earlier time, presented for pain clinic intervention. This study should not, therefore, be considered a study of nerve-block treatment outcome. As noted earlier, the focus of the study is rather on the context in which such treatment is administered. This study is somewhat compromised by the lack of comparability of respondents in the two surveys. Patients who responded to the original survey but *not* to the present follow-up were younger individuals who were more objectively impaired, as evidenced by their decreased ability to bend, but more inclined to rely on their own resources for managing pain as suggested by their lower use of medication. Thus, patients willing to participate in a long-term follow-up survey seem to be older patients who are, perhaps, more entrenched in a "sick-role" lifestyle. The survey results may, therefore, be biased toward an under-reporting of functional gains. In spite of methodologic limitations, the data emphasize the wide range of behaviors affected by chronic pain and argue against simplistic methods for its evaluation and treatment. The continuation over 5 years of rather severe functional and vocational deficits in some of the sample emphasizes the significance of the chronic pain state as a major health problem that affects almost every aspect of daily life. In view of the complexity of psychosocial factors affecting the improvement status of the patient with chronic pain, the present study is strongly supportive of the integrated pain clinic concept. In such a context the evaluation and modification of both the psychological and physical parameters of pain can occur and realistic efforts at rehabilitation be instituted.

SUMMARY

Seventy patients with chronic low back pain not caused by malignancy returned a questionnaire assessing functional status 5 years after treatment with epidural or subarachnoid nerve blocks. A total of 151 patients had been surveyed 3 years earlier in an initial follow-up. Respondents to the present survey were older, better able to bend, and took more medication for pain than nonrespondents. Results revealed a tendency for the gender-associated differences in improvement noted in the initial survey to be maintained, with women showing greater absolute improvement than men, particularly in vocational abilities. Men were somewhat more improved as a group on the current follow-up than on the initial follow-up. Medication usage for pain remained generally unchanged over time, but the number of respondents reporting the need for additional surgical treatments dramatically declined. Results were seen as indicating the need for using multiple, functional criteria in assessing response to treatment and supporting the integrated pain clinic approach for evaluating and modifying the physical and psychosocial factors associated with the chronic pain state.

REFERENCES

1. Arnhoff, F. N., Triplett, H. B., and Pokorney, B. (1977): Follow-up status of patients treated with nerve blocks for low-back pain. *Anesthesiology*, 46:170–178.
2. Barry, P. J. C., and Kendall, P. H. (1962): Corticosteroid infiltration of the extradural space. *Ann. Phys. Med.*, 6:267–273.
3. Cairns, D., Thomas, L., Mooney, V., and Pace, J. B. (1976): A comprehensive treatment approach to chronic low back pain. *Pain*, 2:301–308.
4. Dilke, T. F. W., Burry, H. C., and Grahame, R. (1972): Extradural corticosteroid injection in management of lumbar nerve root compression. *Br. Med. J.*, 2:635–637.
5. Finneson, B. E. (1976): Modulating effect of secondary gain on the low back pain syndrome. In: *Advances in Pain Research and Therapy*, edited by J. J. Bonica and Albe Fessard, pp. 949–952. Raven Press, New York.
6. Fordyce, W. E. (1974): Operant conditioning: An approach to chronic pain. *Curr. Concepts Pain Analg.*, 1:1–11.
7. Fordyce, W. E., Fowler, R. S., Lehmann, J. F., De Lateur, B. J., Sand, P. L., and Trieschmann, R. B. (1973): Operant conditioning in the treatment of chronic pain. *Arch. Phys. Med.*, 54:399–408.
8. Goebert, H. W., Jallo, S. J., Gardner, W. J., et al. (1960): Sciatica: Treatment with epidural injections of procaine and hydrocortisone. *Cleve. Clin. Q.*, 27:191–197.
9. Hammonds, W., Brena, S., and Unikel, I. P. (1977): Compensation for work-related injuries and the rehabilitation of patients with chronic pain. Paper presented at Southern Medical Association, Dallas, Texas.
10. Hulka, B. S., Kupper, L. L., Cassel, J. C., et al. (1971): A method for measuring physicians' awareness of patients concerns. *HSMHA-Health Reports*, 86:741.
11. Ignelzi, R. J., and Sternbach, R. A., and Timmermans, G. (1977): The pain ward follow-up analysis. *Pain*, 3:277–285.
12. Newman, R. I., Seres, J. L., Yospe, L. P., and Garlington, B. (1978): Multi-disciplinary treatment of chronic pain: long-term follow-up of low-back patients. *Pain*, 4:283–292.
13. Rosenthal, R. H., and Murphy, W. (1979): Subjective and objective improvement as related to litigation and financial gain in the treatment of chronic back pain. Paper presented at Southeastern Psychological Association, New Orleans, Louisiana.
14. Sternbach, R. A. (1974): *Pain Patients, Traits and Treatment*. Academic Press, New York.
15. Turner, J., McCreary, C., and Dawson, E. (1978): Functional limitations as predictors of response to treatment for back pain. Paper presented at Second World Congress on Pain, Montreal, Canada.
16. Winnie, A. P., Hartman, J. T., Meyers, H. L., et al. (1972): Pain Clinic II: Intradural and extradural corticosteroids for sciatica. *Anesth. Analg. (Cleve)*, 51:990–999.
17. Wyckoff, M. G., and Chapman, C. R. (1978): A multivariate descriptive study of specific psychologic and sociologic factors present in 100 randomly sampled chronic pain patients. Paper presented at Second World Congress on Pain, Montreal, Canada.

Chronic Low Back Pain, edited by
M. Stanton-Hicks and Robert Boas.
Raven Press, New York © 1982.

Diagnosis of Low Back Pain

John J. Calabro

Department of Rheumatology, Saint Vincent Hospital and Departments of Medicine and Pediatrics, University of Massachusetts Medical School, Worcester, Massachusetts 01604

Chronic low back pain is one of mankind's oldest and most difficult problems. In the United States alone, several million Americans have chronic back problems. Of these, five million are partially disabled whereas another two million are unable to work at all (34).

Why does the low back ache? Clearly, in part, it is the price that humans pay for standing erect. However, there is also a contemporary aspect to chronic back problems. As people become more and more sedentary in an increasingly automated world, doing more work in a sitting position and adding extra pounds of girth, their backs become continuously more vulnerable to injury and osteoporosis. Nevertheless, the lower spine is a marvel of biological engineering. It not only serves as the major conduit for the spinal cord that links the brain with other parts of the body but also furnishes support for the upper portion of the body. In addition, because there are no ribs attached to it, the lower spine has a relatively wide range of motion and, in fact, can be bent to form two-thirds of a circle (34).

CAUSES OF CHRONIC LOW BACK PAIN

It must be clearly understood that low back pain is a symptom and not a disease and that the cause of the pain frequently lies outside of the spine (21). Classification is difficult, as is some of the terminology that is commonly used. The old term *lumbago* should be abandoned, not only because it is confusing but also because it has no diagnostic implications (20). Indeed, the possible causes of chronic low back pain are so numerous that pinpointing the precise one is often a difficult diagnostic challenge. In fact, the physician has to consider everything from poor posture to malignancy (Table 1).

As varied as low back problems may be, up to 80% of those who complain of chronic low back pain are victims of pathomechanical, structural, or functional disorders, such as injury, scoliosis, or poor posture. Lack of exercise also promotes loss of spinal muscle tone and vertebral body demineralization (osteoporosis), as does obesity. The potbelly puts enormous pressure on the spine because as the belly thrusts out, the buttocks push back to offset the extra weight in front and the normal curvature of the spine deepens (34). For women, the problem becomes especially prominent in the last months of pregnancy when many suffer chronic back pain.

TABLE 1. *Classification of chronic low back pain*

Major Causes	Examples
Structural/functional disorders	Scoliosis/poor posture
Pathomechanical disorders	Fracture, dislocation
Root compression	Herniated disk, degenerative disk disease
Infection	Pott's disease
Metabolic disorders	Primary osteoporosis
Neoplastic diseases	Multiple myeloma, metastatic malignancy
Referred Pain	Inflammatory or other chronic disorders of the pelvis or abdomen
Rheumatic disorders	Ankylosing spondylitis, Reiter's syndrome, primary fibrositis

DIAGNOSIS

The diagnosis of low back pain depends on a careful history, a thorough physical examination, and routine laboratory and X-ray studies (20). Occasionally, a precise diagnosis may be achieved only by repeated examination and special tests. Only then can logical management be instituted. For most back problems, the history often provides the most critical clues.

History

This should include the patient's age, sex, and race, the socioeconomic and past medical history, a general review of systems, the family history, as well as the type of work and daily activities of the patient. Backache can affect almost anyone, the young and the old and people of all classes and occupations. Age is a useful consideration in diagnosis. In children, for example, sprains, injury, spondylolysis, spondylolisthesis, and scoliosis are frequent causes whereas herniated disk is rare (18). On the other hand, the major causes of back pain in the elderly are degenerative (spondylosis, osteoarthritis, and diffuse idiopathic skeletal hyperostosis), neoplastic (multiple myeloma and metastases from malignancy), and metabolic (osteoporosis, osteomalacia, chondrocalcinosis, and Paget's disease) (3). In postmenopausal women a major cause of chronic back pain is primary osteoporosis. In young men, however, the leading causes are injury and herniated disk, but if the problem is systemic, then ankylosing spondylitis and Reiter's syndrome become major possibilities (7). The family history is especially relevant because many disorders such as scoliosis, ochronosis, ankylosing spondylitis (33), and Reiter's syndrome (8,36) run in families.

The young man with ankylosing spondylitis usually has difficulty sleeping because nocturnal pain is a characteristic feature of this disorder. The patient with spondylitis also awakens with early morning stiffness that gradually eases as he moves about and increases his activity. In fact, these two features—early morning stiffness and nocturnal pain—are such typical manifestations of ankylosing spondylitis that their absence seriously suggests consideration of other diagnoses (13). Associated fever and chills suggest infection, not necessarily localized in the spine but perhaps referred to the back from a neighboring organ. Chronic pyelonephritis and pelvic inflammatory disease are common causes of referred pain to the back. Even aneurysms or peripheral vascular disease may give rise to backache or symptoms resembling sciatica (21).

Other major considerations are the source and character of the pain (20). Involvement of a single spinal nerve root produces a sensation that is confined to the peripheral dermatome of that nerve root. The onset of symptoms is acute. The pain is sharp, lancinating, and accompanied by paresthesia and numbness. Pain produced by stimuli within deep skeletal structures, such as muscle, ligaments, fascia, and periosteum, is quite different. Such pain is insidious in onset. It is vaguely localized, aching in character, radiating over greater distances, and relatively prolonged in duration.

Is the pain steady or intermittent in character? If intermittent, at what times of the day does it recur? Pain at night or in the early morning suggests arthritis. Pain related to certain activities or movements suggests injury, strain, or disk disease. Is the pain aggravated by bending or by sneezing or coughing, as in disk disease? Is it relieved by rest or activity or by massage, heat, or a particular medication? For example, back pain from ankylosing spondylitis is so consistently relieved by indomethacin or phenylbutazone that if neither of these drugs eases discomfort, the diagnosis should be seriously challenged (6).

Physical Examination

The general physical examination may disclose signs suggesting certain diagnoses. An abnormal prostatic examination in a man with low back pain may be the only clinical clue to vertebral metastases from prostatic malignancy. Skin tags or pedunculated tumors may indicate the presence of neurofibromatosis whereas excessive port wine or birth marks may be associated with underlying bony abnormalities, such as spinal bifida (19). Darkened sclerae or skin may be features of ochronosis whereas onycholysis should suggest spondylitis from either psoriasis or Reiter's syndrome (10).

The examination of the back should be conducted in an orderly manner (21). More errors in diagnosis are made from want of proper examination than for any other reason (21). Always observe the patient's stance and posture. A minimal degree of lumbar lordosis is normal. However, the normal lumbar lordosis is lost and flattening results when muscle spasm is present. Palpate for areas of tenderness, spasm, or other abnormalities.

When examining the back, flexion, lateral bending, and extension are the most important motions to evaluate. Limited back motion can usually be detected by these maneuvers. Normal back motion implies that the underlying disorder may be functional or that the origin of the problem may be elsewhere, perhaps even in the hips, knees, or feet.

There are a number of special tests, too numerous to describe but carefully outlined elsewhere, that can be useful in differential diagnosis (19–21). Straight-leg raising often reproduces radicular pain suggesting nerve-root irritation. A positive Schober's test is common in ankylosing spondylitis, but it is nonspecific and diagnosis depends on the disclosure of other typical features, such as sacroiliac tenderness and diminished chest expansion (Table 2) (7).

In our changing society, the prevalence of low back pain is constantly being influenced directly by various social and psychological factors. Consequently, disclosure of potential psychic factors has become a necessary part of the clinical evaluation (20). Moreover, it must be remembered that the clinical presentation may often be clouded and confused by emotional overtones (21).

Laboratory and X-ray Studies

The presence of acute phase reactants, for example, an elevated erythrocyte sedimentation rate (ESR), supports the diagnosis of a systemic rheumatic disorder, such as ankylosing spondylitis or Reiter's syndrome. On the other hand, a normal ESR suggests that the problem is pathomechanical or functional (27). The clinical setting should direct the clinician to special studies, such as bone marrow aspiration for a diagnosis of multiple myeloma or testing for the HLA-B27 antigen if spondylitis or Reiter's syndrome is suspected (35).

Evaluation of a low back problem is not complete without radiologic studies (20). With anteroposterior and lateral views of the lumbar spine taken with the patient in a supine position, details of the vertebral bodies, sacrum, and the sacroiliac and intervertebral joints should reveal significant abnormalities, including defects

TABLE 2. *Clinical test to detect early ankylosing spondylitis*

Test	Method	Interpretation
Fingers to floor	Patient bends forward with his knees straight (Fig. 1) and distance from fingertips to floor is measured.	Inability to touch close to the floor suggests lumbar involvement.
Schober test	While the patient is standing erect, make a mark on the spine at the level of the iliac crests and another mark 10 cm directly above. Patient then bends forward maximally and the distance between the two marks is measured.	An increase of less than 5 cm indicates early lumbar involvement.
Chest expansion	Measure maximum chest expansion at nipple line.	Chest expansion of less than 3 cm is a clue to early costovertebral involvement.
Sacroiliac compression	Exert direct compression over sacroiliac joints (Fig.2).	Local tenderness suggests sacroiliac involvement, which may otherwise be asymptomatic.

in the neural arch and facets. Occasionally, oblique and other views may be necessary. There may also be a need for special procedures, such as myelography, electromyography, discography, radioactive scanning, or needle aspiration and biopsy.

RHEUMATIC DISORDERS

I would like to devote this segment to a consideration of ankylosing spondylitis, Reiter's syndrome, and primary fibrositis, not only because back discomfort is common to each of these disorders but also because early diagnosis is often difficult.

Ankylosing Spondylitis

The precise etiology of ankylosing spondylitis is uncertain. Nevertheless, the recent disclosure of an unusually high frequency (90%) of the inherited antigen HLA-B27 in patients and their relatives compared with only 6 to 9% in healthy Caucasian controls provides overwhelming evidence of a genetic predisposition in this disorder (4,9,29).

Ankylosing spondylitis is a systemic rheumatic disorder primarily found in young men that is characterized by inflammation of the sacroiliac and spinal apophyseal (synovial) joints. Consequently, low back pain is a frequent presenting symptom, although the disease can begin in peripheral joints and in rare instances even with acute iridocyclitis (6,7). Early diagnosis, therefore, rests on the recognition of these three modes of onset and is confirmed by a few simple tests that can be performed in the office as part of the routine physical examination (Table 2). These tests facilitate detection of early disease at a time when management poses the fewest problems.

Involvement of the lumbar spine is present when the patient cannot touch the floor while keeping his knees extended (Fig. 1). A positive Schober's test and lumbar flattening caused by paravertebral muscle spasm may be present as well. Reduced chest expansion is a clue to the presence of asymptomatic costovertebral involvement whereas sacroiliac compression helps to detect sacroiliitis (Fig. 2). The ESR is elevated in most patients as are other acute phase reactants. Presence of the HLA-B27 antigen is perhaps the single best laboratory clue. Its absence, however, does not preclude the diagnosis.

The diagnosis of ankylosing spondylitis is confirmed by X-ray. However, it does not depend on disclosure of the classic "bamboo" spine with its prominent syndesmophytes and diffuse paraspinal ligamentous calcification (Fig. 3),which is clearly a late manifestation that is found in a minority of patients with severe and progressive disease. The most characteristic early findings occur in the sacroiliac joints, initially with subchondral erosions and sclerosis (Fig. 4), and later with progressive narrowing of the joints that is typically symmetrical.

A technique that provides a craniocaudal axial view of the sacroiliac joints has recently been reported (14). It can apparently disclose ventral ankylosis of joints that is not visible or is only suspected on anteroposterior views. Also scintigraphy

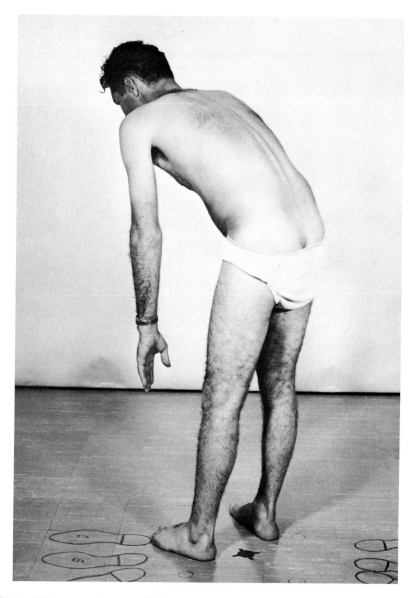

FIG. 1. Patient bends forward with knees straight and is able to reach only to the knees, indicating early lumbar involvement. Minimal lumbar flattening is also present.

or quantitative scanning techniques may be beneficial in early cases in which routine sacroiliac X-rays are normal (16,23). However, with this approach, the skill and experience of the interpreter are obviously important, as is the clinical input of the patient being evaluated. Indeed, false-positive scanning values have been reported in patients with metabolic bone disease and with structural abnormalities of the low

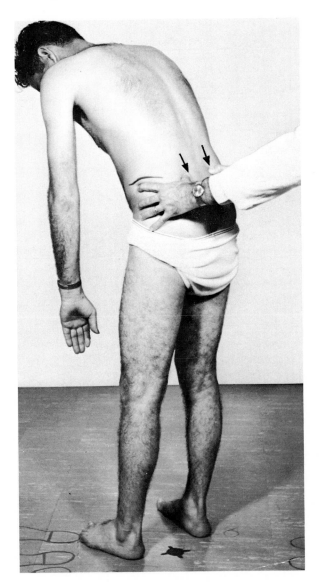

FIG. 2. Direct compression is applied to the sacroiliac joints *(arrows)*. Local tenderness or gluteal pain reveals sacroiliitis, which may be asymptomatic in the early stages.

back (16). Early abnormalities of the lumbar spine include vertebral squaring and demineralization (Fig. 5). Minimal ligamentous calcification and one or two evolving syndesmophytes may also be present.

Syndesmophytes should not be confused with osteophytes. The latter are found frequently in the middle-aged and almost universally in the elderly but are usually

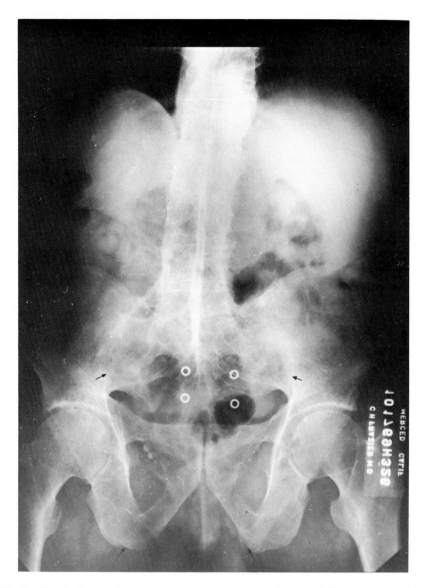

FIG. 3. Classic "bamboo" spine with prominent syndesmophytes and diffuse paraspinal ligamentous calcification and fused sacroiliac joints *(arrows)*, as seen in advanced disease.

asymptomatic. Consequently, if X-ray examination reveals that a patient with backache has osteophytes, the two may not necessarily be related, and other causes should be considered before accepting the diagnosis of osteoarthritis.

Diffuse idiopathic skeletal hyperostosis (DISH), or Forestier's disease, occurs primarily in men over the age of 50 and resembles ankylosing spondylitis both

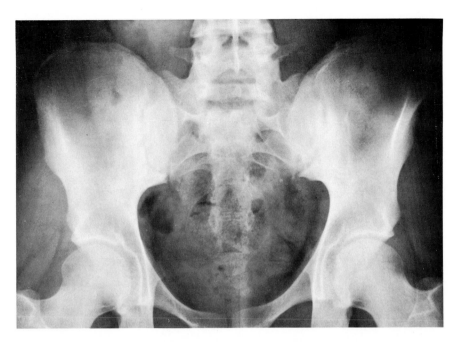

FIG. 4. Pelvic X-ray discloses "pseudowidening" of the sacroiliac joints from subchondral erosions and sclerosis that are more prominent on the iliac side.

clinically and on X-ray. Patients with DISH may have spinal pain, stiffness, and loss of motion that develops insidiously (25). Radiological findings include ossification of the anterior and lateral ligaments that most often occurs in the cervical and lower thoracic region. However, in DISH, the disk spaces and the sacroiliac and apophyseal joints are not involved, and vertebral squaring and demineralization are not present (25).

One of the most important disorders from which ankylosing spondylitis must be distinguished is a herniated lumbar disk. In the latter affliction, the ESR is normal, and the HLA-B27 antigen is not usually present. The only certain way to diagnose a herniated disk is to document the defect with myelography or CT scanning.

Juvenile Ankylosing Spondylitis

Until recently, it has not been appreciated that pauciarticular arthritis of childhood may precede and herald the development of spondylitis by years (11). Children in whom ankylosing spondylitis subsequently develops are usually boys with arthritis involving only a few lower limb joints and a disease onset in late childhood (1,11,28). In all but 4 of 52 children presenting with a peripheral arthritis who were subsequently diagnosed as having juvenile ankylosing spondylitis, the onset of peripheral arthritis occurred after age 8 (1). The mean age of onset was 12 years whereas the mean age at the time of sacroiliitis disclosure was 18 years; thus, there was a mean

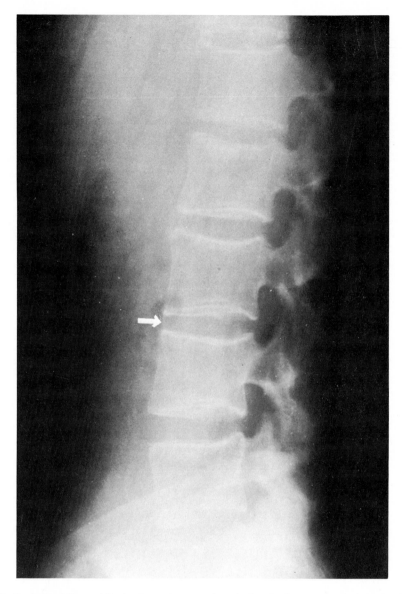

FIG. 5. Lateral X-ray of the lumbar spine reveals typical early changes that include demineralization and squaring of vertebral bodies and ligamentous calcification seen only at L_3 to L_4 *(arrow).*

lapse of 6 years between the onset of peripheral arthritis and the development of back complaints. Laboratory clues include negative tests for both rheumatoid factor and antinuclear antibodies and a positive test for B27 antigen. Consequently, in differentiating children with ankylosing spondylitis from those with rheumatoid arthritis, HLA typing can be of great value (7).

Spondylitis in Women

Women with ankylosing spondylitis appear to have milder or atypical disease that may go unrecognized for years (7). A clinical and radiographic study of 98 patients with spondylitis was undertaken to evaluate differences in men and women who had the disease (24). Atypical clinical manifestations, seen more frequently in the 18 women patients than in the 80 men, included (a) older age of disease onset, (b) higher frequency of initial and subsequent peripheral joint involvement, (c) more frequent cervical spine symptoms, and (d) a milder disease course. X-ray differences in the women include (a) a higher frequency of cervical spine abnormalities, (b) a greater tendency for combined cervical spine and sacroiliac changes with sparing of the intervening thoracic and lumbar spine, and (c) more frequent and severe osteitis pubis. Moreover, spondylitis in women evolves more slowly than in men so that typical X-ray and clinical features may take an average of 10 years to appear (17).

Ankylosing spondylitis in women should not be confused with osteitis condensans ilii, a syndrome particularly common in postpartum women that may be related to the strain that delivery imposes on the sacroiliac joints. It is characterized by unilateral or bilateral triangular bony sclerosis of the lower ilium (Fig. 6). Although low back pain is a common feature of osteitis condensans ilii, patients do not develop limitation of spinal movement, X-ray evidence of spondylitis, or the progressive course seen in ankylosing spondylitis (30). Furthermore, as shown by HLA typing, the frequency of the B27 antigen in osteitis condensans ilii is comparable to that of controls (15,26). Consequently, osteitis condensans ilii is not a variant of ankylosing spondylitis in women, as has been so often suggested in the past.

Primary osteoporosis, which may also be mistaken for ankylosing spondylitis, is one of the more common causes of backache in the middle-aged and elderly and is particularly prominent in postmenopausal women. Typically, back pain is worse when the patient is up and about and is relieved by rest (27). Examination often reveals an increased roundness of the back and loss of height. There are characteristic X-ray changes, including demineralization, wedging, and collapse of vertebrae most frequent in the lower thoracic but also in the lumbar spine.

Reiter's Syndrome

The symptom complex known as Reiter's syndrome has recently emerged from a disorder of relative oscurity to one of great fascination and importance (12). This has clearly evolved from recent recognition of the striking association between Reiter's syndrome and the presence of the HLA-B27 antigen (9).

One of the more common systemic forms of arthritis of young men, Reiter's syndrome occurs most frequently between the ages of 20 and 40 years (10). The syndrome is rare in women, and presentation is often atypical (31). Although

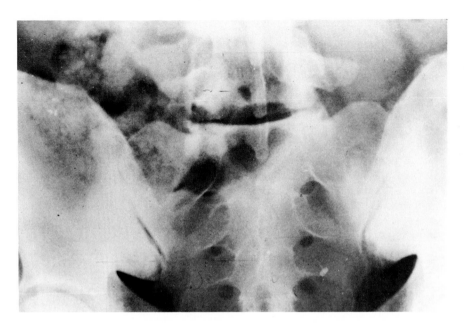

FIG. 6. Sclerosis of the iliac bone is present as a triangular density adjacent to the sacroiliac joints. The sacrum and sacroiliac joints are not involved. Osteitis condensans ilii may affect one or both sides but should not be confused with the sclerosis of ankylosing spondylitis.

traditionally regarded as a self-limiting triad of nonspecific urethritis, conjunctivitis, and arthritis, it is now apparent that Reiter's syndrome is neither self-limiting nor a triad (9,10). In fact, recurrence or chronicity is reported in at least half of the patients, and the triad is often incomplete in patients who clearly have the disease (2,10). Key diagnosis features, often not sought for because of their painless nature, include (a) hyperkeratotic nail and skin lesions (Fig. 7), which bear a striking resemblance to psoriasis, (b) circinate balanitis, (c) superficial ulcerations of the oral mucosa (Fig. 8), and (d) a geographic tongue. The arthritis is florid and distinctly the most disabling manifestation. Swelling tends to be asymmetrical and usually involves only a few joints, especially knees, ankles, and feet. Low back and sacroiliac tenderness may also occur. When back complaints become chronic, patients should be monitored closely for the development of Reiter's spondylitis.

Laboratory findings can be helpful in making the diagnosis. The ESR is usually elevated, and a moderate degree of neutrophilic leucocytosis and normochromic anemia may be present. The B27 antigen is present in 63 to 96% of patients whether the back is involved or not (2,5,21,22). X-ray examination shows that sacroiliac abnormalities are often unilateral or asymmetric (Fig. 9) and therefore quite dissimilar to the symmetrical configuration seen in ankylosing spondylitis. Also, unlike those seen in ankylosing spondylitis (Fig. 10), the syndesmophytes of Reiter's spondylitis tend to be asymmetric and nonmarginal (Fig. 11).

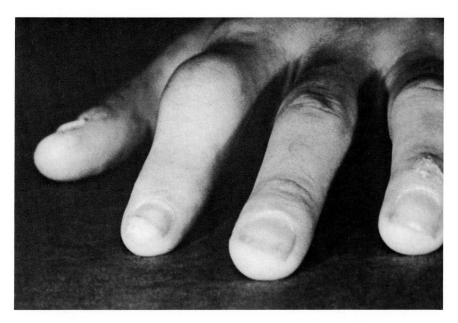

FIG. 7. Note onychylosis of the nail of the second finger, an accumulation of white, waxy material under the distal end of the nail plate. The hyperkeratotic lesion at the distal end of the fourth finger bears a striking similarity to pustular psoriasis. There is also swelling of a single proximal interphalangeal joint.

Perhaps the disorder that is the most difficult to differentiate from Reiter's syndrome is psoriatic arthritis (10). This is because the lesions of pustular psoriasis and the hyperkeratotic cutaneous lesions of Reiter's syndrome may be indistinguishable both clinically and histologically. In psoriasis, however, urethritis and conjunctivitis do not occur and the oral mucosa is rarely involved. Also, nail pitting—a frequent finding in psoriatic arthritis— does not occur in Reiter's syndrome.

Primary Fibrositis

Fibrositis, also known as fibromyositis, myofibrositis, and fibromyalgia, is a common form of nonarticular rheumatism characterized by diffuse aches and stiffness of muscles, ligaments, tendon insertions, subcutaneous tissues, and bony prominences. The syndrome can be classified as (a) *primary* when no demonstrable cause or underlying systemic disease is present and when all findings, including the ESR and X-rays, are normal, and (b) *secondary* to other chronic illness, such as the rheumatic diseases, bone disorders, infections, and malignancy.

Primary fibrositis occurs most frequently in young and middle-aged women, although it is not confined to this group. The cause is unknown. Muscle and tendon inflammation, implied by the term *fibromyositis* has never been demonstrated. In

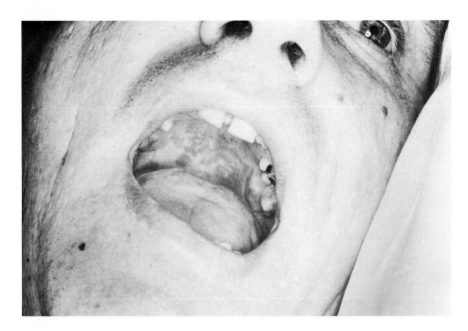

FIG. 8. Superficial, painless ulcerations of the palate caused by Reiter's syndrome.

fact, the finding of inflammation either on physical examination or by laboratory parameters would rule against the diagnosis.

The onset of symptoms is rarely acute, usually described as "hurting for months or years," with frequent flares and remissions. Patients complain of musculoskeletal pain and stiffness that is usually worse in the morning but occasionally in the evening, particularly after a hectic working day. Symptoms are often intensified by cold and damp weather, inactivity, excessive unaccustomed physical activity, fatigue, and mental tension. Symptoms are lessened by warm weather, activity, heat, massage, and recreation. Most patients sleep poorly, and many complain of chronic fatigue, tension, headache, or emotional distress.

Examination of the joints reveals no abnormalities except for the presence of trigger points, points of excessive local tenderness that are found at precisely predictable symmetrical sites (32). Common trigger points are the elbows, shoulders, medial border of the scapulae, cervical, thoracic, and lumbosacral areas of the spine, sacroiliac joints, medial fat pad of the knees, and the second costochondral junctions. These sites are normally somewhat tender so that excessive pressure during palpation should be avoided. Muscle spasm may be marked in some patients. Occasionally, pea- to plum-sized fibro-fatty nodules can be palpated. Recently, fibrositis patients have been shown to have EEG abnormalities of non-REM (non-rapid eye movement) sleep. In fact, experimental disturbances in non-REM sleep of healthy volunteers has produced tenderness in the usual trigger points (32).

Fibrositis should not be confused with psychogenic rheumatism. The latter has a bizarre pattern of rheumatic symptoms regulated by the patient's psychic status

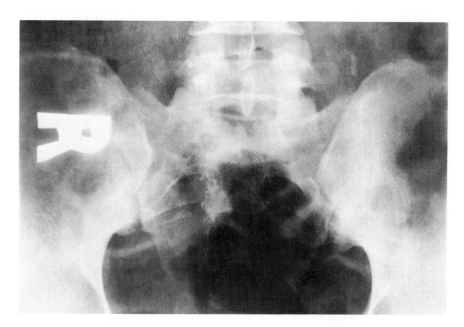

FIG. 9. Sacroiliac abnormalities in Reiter's syndrome tend to be asymmetric: the right sacro-iliac joint is narrowed but the left is completely fused.

rather than exogenous factors, such as weather and activity. Moreover, typical trigger points are not found in patients with psychogenic rheumatism.

CONCLUSIONS

Chronic low back pain is a strikingly common ailment affecting millions of Americans of all ages. The possible causes are numerous and frequently originate from sources outside the spine. Nevertheless, diagnosis is possible in the majority of cases but depends on an orderly evaluation, including a careful history, a thorough physical examination, and routine laboratory and X-ray studies. Occasionally, the diagnosis can only be clarified by special studies and/or repeated evaluations of the patient.

Ankylosing spondylitis, Reiter's syndrome, and primary fibrositis are three of the more common rheumatic disorders that are often difficult to diagnose. The early recognition of ankylosing spondylitis rests on awareness that there are three distinct modes of onset and that the disease can evolve differently in both children and women than it does in men. Key diagnostic features of Reiter's syndrome, often not sought for because of their painless nature, include hyperkeratotic skin and nail changes, circinate balanitis, and superficial ulcerations of the oral mucosa. Although the presence of the HLA-B27 antigen is a useful diagnostic clue for both ankylosing spondylitis and Reiter's syndrome, it should be clear that each can occur in the absence of this antigen. Primary fibrositis is a common form of nonarticular rheu-

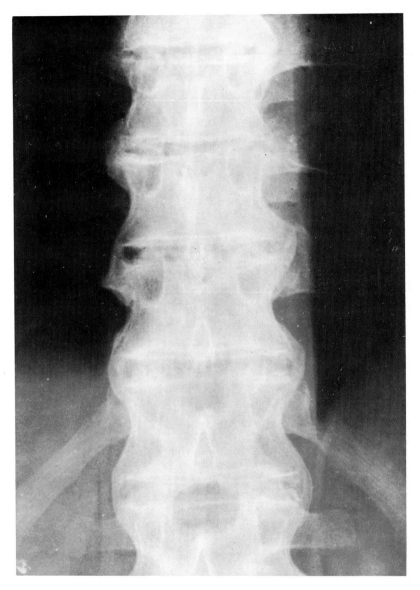

FIG. 10. The syndesmophytes of typical ankylosing spondylitis tend to be marginal and symmetric.

matism that is characterized by the presence of typical trigger points. Diagnosis depends on awareness of the clinical profile of the syndrome, normal laboratory and X-ray findings, and careful observation to rule out secondary causes.

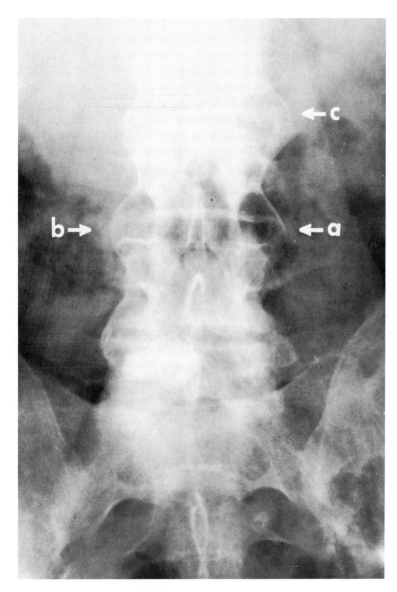

FIG. 11. The syndesmophytes of Reiter's spondylitis are usually asymmetric and nonmarginal. They may appear in various evolutionary stages: first as a minimal linear projection *(a)*, then as bridging across contiguous vertebrae *(b)*, and finally as thick, tubular bridging *(c)*.

REFERENCES

1. Ansell, B. M. (1977): Ankylosing spondylitis. *Arthritis Rheum.*, 20 (Supp):414–415.
2. Arnett, F. C., McClusky, O. E., Schacter, B. Z., and Lordon, R. E. (1976): Incomplete Reiter's syndrome: Discriminating features and HL-A W27 in diagnosis. *Ann. Int. Med.*, 84:8–12.
3. Bandilla, K. K. (1977): Back pain: Osteoarthritis. *J. Am. Geriatr. Soc.*, 25:62–66.

4. Brewerton, D. A., Caffrey, M., Hart, F. D., James, D. C. O., Nicholls, A., Sturrock, R. D. (1973): Ankylosing spondylitis and HL-A 27. *Lancet*, 1:904–907.
5. Brewerton, D. A., Caffrey, M., Nicholls, A., Water, D., Oates, J. K., and James, D. C. O. (1973): Reiter's disease and HL-A 27. *Lancet*, 2:996–998.
6. Calabro, J. J., 1968: An appraisal of the medical and surgical management of ankylosing spondylitis. *Clin. Orthop.*, 60:125–148.
7. Calabro, J. J. (1977): Early diagnosis and management of ankylosing spondylitis. *Med. Times*, 105:80–96.
8. Calabro, J. J., Calabro, J. A., Boland, D. M., Stanton, G. F., and Yunus, M. (1977): Reiter's syndrome in siblings. *JAMA*, 238:2484.
9. Calabro, J. J., Castor, C. W., Cohen, A. S., Clayton, M. L., Decker, J. L., Ferguson, R. H., Gordon, D., Hench, P. K., Johnson, R. L., Klinenberg, J. R., Myers, A. R., Schaller, J. G., Schmid, F. R., Tourtellotte, C. D., Winchester, R. J., and Zurier, R. B. (1978): Twenty-third rheumatism review. *Arthritis Rheum.*, 21 (Suppl):R38–R46.
10. Calabro, J. J., and Garg, S. L. (1974): Reiter's syndrome. In: *Practice of medicine, Vol. 5* edited by G. B. Bluhm, pp. 1–20. Harper & Row Publishers, Inc., Hagerstown, Maryland.
11. Calabro, J. J., Holgerson, W. B., Sonpal, G. M., and Khoury, M. I. (1976): Juvenile rheumatoid arthritis: A general review and report of 100 patients observed for 15 years. *Semin. Arthritis Rheum.*, 5:257–298.
12. Calin, A. (1977): Reiter's syndrome. *Med. Clin. N. Am.*, 61:365–376.
13. Calin, A., Porta, J., Fries, J. F., Schurman, D. J. (1977): Clinical history as a screening test for ankylosing spondylitis. *JAMA*, 237:2613–2613.
14. Dory, M. S., Francois, R. J. (1978): Craniocaudal axial view of sacroiliac joint. *Am. J. Roentgenol.*, 130:1125–1131.
15. Ercilla, M. G., Grancos, M. A., Breysse, Y., Alonso, G., Vives, J., Castillo, R., and Rotes-Querol, J. (1977): HLA antigens in Forestier's disease, ankylosing spondylitis, and polyarthrosis of the hands. *J. Rheumatol.*, 4 (Suppl):89–93.
16. Goldberg, R. P., Genant, H. F., Shimshak, R., and Shames, D. (1978): Applications and limitations of quantitative sacroiliac joint scintigraphy. *Radiology*, 128:683–686.
17. Hill, H. F. H., Hill, A. G. S., and Bodmer, J. G. (1976): Clinical diagnosis of ankylosing spondylitis in women and relation to presence of HLA-B27. *Ann. Rheumat. Dis.*, 35:267–270.
18. Hoppenfeld, S. (1977): Back pain. *Pediatric Clin. N. Am.*, 24:881–887.
19. Hoppenfeld, S. (1976): Physical examination of the lumbar spine. In: *Physical Examination of the Spine and Extremities*, edited by S. Hoppenfeld, pp. 237–263. Appleton-Century-Crofts, New York.
20. Levine, D. G. (1979): The painful low back. In: *Arthritis and Allied Conditions*, edited by D. J. McCarty, pp. 1044–1097. Grune & Stratton, New York.
21. Macnab, I. (1977): *Backache*. Williams & Wilkins Co., Baltimore, Maryland.
22. Morris, R., Metzger, A. L., Bluestone, R., and Terasaki, P. I. (1974): HL-A W27—a clue to the diagnosis and pathogenesis of Reiter's syndrome. *N. Engl. J. Med.*, 290:554–556.
23. Namey, T. C., McIntyre, J., Buse, M., and LeRoy, E. C. (1977): Nucleographic studies of axial spondarthritides. *Arthritis Rheum.*, 20:1058–1064.
24. Resnick, D., Dwosh, I. L., Goergen, T. G., Shapiro, R. F., Utsinger, P. D., Wiesner, K. B., and Bryan, B. L. (1976): Clinical and radiographic abnormalities in ankylosing spondylitis—comparison of men and women. *Radiology*, 119:293–297.
25. Resnick, D., Shapiro, R. F., Wiesner, K. B., Niwayama, G., Utsinger, P. D., and Shaul, S. R. (1978): Diffuse idiopathic skeletal hyperostosis (DISH) (ankylosing hyperostosis of Forestier and Rotes-Querol). *Semin. Arthritis Rheum.*, 7:153–187.
26. Rosenthal, M., Bahouse, I., Muller, W. (1977): Increased frequency of HLA B8 in hyperostotic spondylosis. *J. Rheumatol.*, 4 (Suppl):89–93.
27. Sarkin, T. L. (1977): Backache in the aged, *S. Afr. Med. J.*, 51:418–420.
28. Schaller, J. G., Ochs, H. D., Thomas, E. D., Nisperos, B., Feigl, P., and Wedgwood, R. (1976): Histocompatibility antigens in childhood-onset arthritis. *J. Pediatr.*, 88:926–930.
29. Schlosstein, L., Terasaki, P. I., Bluestone, R., Pearson, C. M. (1973): High association of the HL-A antigen, W27, with ankylosing spondylitis, *New Engl. J. Med.*, 288:704–706.
30. Singal, D. P., de Bosset, P., Gordon, D. A., Smythe, M. A., Urowitz, M. B., and Koehler, B. E. (1977): HLA antigens in osteitis condensans ilii and ankylosing spondylitis. *J. Rheumatol. (Supp 3)*, 4:105–108.

31. Smith, D. L., Bennett, R. M., and Regan, M. G. (1980): Reiter's disease in women. *Arthritis Rheum.*, 23:335–340.
32. Smythe, H. A., and Maldofsky, H. (1977): Two contributions to understanding of the "fibrositis syndrome". *Bull. Rheumat. Dis.*, 28:928–931.
33. Strosberg, J. M., Allen, F. H., Calabro, J. J., Harris, E. D. Jr.(1975): Ankylosing spondylitis in a large kindred: Clinical and genetic studies. *Tissue Antigens*, 5:205–212.
34. Toufexis, A. (1980): That aching back! *Time Magazine*, 116:30–38.
35. Woodrow, J. C. (1977): Histocompatibility antigens and rheumatic diseases. *Semin. Arthritis Rheum.*, 6:257–276.
36. Yunus, M., Masi, A. T., Calabro, J. J., Miller, K. A., and Yunis, E. J. (1980): A high familial association of Reiter's syndrome among B27 positive first degree relatives. *Arthritis Rheum.*, 23:766.

Chronic Low Back Pain, edited by
M. Stanton-Hicks and Robert Boas.
Raven Press, New York © 1982.

Pathomechanics and Treatment of Low Back Pain and Sciatica
An Abbreviated Overview After a Lecture

Alf Nachemson

Department of Orthopaedic Surgery, Sahlgren Hospital, S-413 45 Göteborg, Sweden

Low back pain is a universal disease. It is also a condition that is always associated with various psychological factors. It is no accident that having a strong back is considered to be a sign of strength and that to have a normally functioning back is perhaps more important to us as individuals in a modern society than for the Neanderthal man (8). As a corollary, therefore, as soon as one is afflicted with back pain, one is immediately put at a disadvantage and made to feel weak. Likewise, depending on one's own psychological makeup, he or she will manifest the symptoms of back pain to a greater or lesser degree.

It is common fallacy that because human beings walk on their hind legs, they are more susceptible candidates for low back pain. However, we know that all animals with spines have back pain. Studies carried out in different centers around the world have demonstrated this fact. One statistic that is unquestionable is that at some time in life, 80% of human beings will have back pain to a varying degree, but of this group, only a small percentage will end up with a chronic back pain syndrome (39).

Unfortunately, many of our problems as professionals are complicated by the fact that we do not speak the same language. The osteopath uses a different vocabulary from that of the orthopedic surgeon, which again is different from that of the acupuncturist, which is naturally different from that of the chiropractor, and so on. Nevertheless, all these diverse practitioners seem to achieve about the same degree of success in their management of this syndrome. A common language would certainly improve the dialogue between these groups. For example, back "insufficiency" is often used to describe a tiredness of the back; "lumbago" is a term used to describe a pain at the base of the back; and "sciatica" is a term used to describe a pain that radiates down one leg or the other. It is obvious that agreement on the meaning of these terms would be a major triumph. Likewise, the adjective "acute" should be used only where there is in fact an acute onset of symptoms; the term "chronic" should apply only where the symptoms have been extant for more than 3 months; and "subacute" should be used to refer to the slow onset of symptoms that are of less than 3 months' duration.

One should look at back pain systematically by describing the clinical components, the bioengineering components, or the biological components. If it is recognized that this is a self-limiting disease, then over 70% of affected individuals
can be expected to get over their acute attack within 3 weeks of its onset whereas
90% will be rid of their symptoms within 2 months. However, the individual's
occupation will have a lot to do with the magnitude of the symptoms. Obviously,
the manual worker will register more pain complaints than his white-collar counterpart because there are mechanical factors that definitely prevent this individual
from carrying on his or her occupation as long as the symptoms are exacerbated
by this sort of activity. However, there are other occupations that aggravate back
pain, most notably driving, whether it be a truck or a car (14).

What means do we have for diagnosis? What do X-rays tell us? One can draw
almost any subjective interpretation from looking at a series of X-rays. There are
no consistent radiological findings associated with injury of the back that can lead
one to the etiological cause of back pain. Features such as single disk narrowing,
subluxation, and facet tropism, seen in one or more lumbar vertebrae, might all be
causes of back pain and yet, just as often, these radiological features are present
in individuals who have no pain whatsoever. In order to stress this point, let us
consider single disk narrowing. Magora, who wrote several epidemiologically important papers that were published in the *Scandinavian Journal of Rehabilitation
Medicine* from 1975 onwards, has demonstrated that single disk degeneration occurs
more often in people who have never had back pain. Yet, this single piece of
objective evidence is responsible for much of the surgery in various parts of the
world that involves spinal fusion and other large operations on the back. Another
radiological finding that has questionable relevance to back pain is spondylolysis.

However, now there are distinctive radiological findings, which are described
by Steinberg elsewhere in this book. Such findings are multiple disk narrowing,
osteoporosis, and spondylolisthesis, although spondylolisthesis by itself does not
necessarily mean that the individual will have back pain. The natural history of
spondylolisthesis is unknown, and although it is not necessarily associated with
back pain, its presence does mean that the individual is at increased risk of suffering
back pain at some time in his or her life.

Another radiological finding that may be associated with back pain is the "too
straight back," that is, the man who in his youth had osteochondritis, or Scheuer-
mann's disease, of the lumbar spine, which results in a poor increase in the height
of the vertebral body relative to the increase in the height of the arch. Such individuals probably need vocational guidance during their growth period, and one
should continue to provide guidance during their twenties in order to forestall the
onset of back pain symptoms later in life.

Let us look at the possible areas where back pain might arise. The motion segments
of the vertebral column contain many different structures. Of course, muscles move
these structures, but so far, no one has been able to demonstrate any pathoanatomical
changes in these muscles, except those changes relative to the denervation that can

accompany disk herniation. Such changes are consistent with nerve root involvement and are no different from those changes seen with any disease that produces denervation. Fibrositis as a pathological entity does not exist: at least, there are no histological changes that lend support to such a condition. Whether ligamentous ruptures exist is also open to question.

The facet joint is another structure on which attention has been focused during recent years. In fact, there probably is what might be considered a facet joint syndrome, although this is poorly described. The typical patient is a younger female with an acute onset of back pain, as contrasted to the older male with a slower onset. This has been demonstrated in controlled studies by O'Brien and his coworkers in Oswestry. We do know that radiological changes exist in facet joints. They occur late and are generally secondary to actual disk degeneration. It is apparent that first there is a pathoanatomical disintegration of the disk leading to mechanical disturbances, and then secondary phenomena involving other structures in this area are seen. However, we do not know what the normal radiological appearance of the facet joint actually is. Unfortunately, it will probably never be known since X-ray studies of these joints give rise to much radiation, and thus no human ethics committee would allow this type of screening nowadays.

It is well-known that aging results in osseous encroachment on the spinal canal. This is termed spinal stenosis. It is also known that from the beginning, the size of the canal is important. Ramani found that individuals who underwent operations for disk herniations had smaller canals than normal. This has recently been corroborated by Porter and collaborators using ultrasound techniques (for a description of this method, see ref. 30). Ultrasound has proved to be a useful tool for measuring the dimensions of the spinal canal. It is noninvasive, and one can obtain a rapid measurement of the approximate dimensions of the human canal. Whether or not this information will be important to the understanding and management of low back pain syndromes remains to be seen. However, it may prove to be of great significance for industrial back trouble.

Having ultrasound pictures of both symptomatic and asymptomatic spines to illustrate the above points would be useful. There are obvious potential difficulties with any screening technique, particularly one that will inevitably select individuals for a particular occupation. Workplace changes should, however, also be instituted.

Crush injuries of the vertebrae can give rise to back pain, even when no obvious fracture exists. There may be microfractures of the trabeculae; such fractures are not obvious with any radiological technique. Although these fractures cannot be seen with the naked eye, the fact that they may be associated with back pain has been brought forward as evidence by Hansson on the basis of laboratory studies (11) and by Troup who, during a 3-year period, followed some 800 industrial workers who had injured themselves as a result of a fall. These workers had a much longer absence and recurrence rate because of back pain than those with other injuries.

The disk still remains a central point of interest, not only because mechanical derangement of a disk disturbs the whole motion segment but also because of many other factors. In 98% of the cases, low back pain precedes disk herniation and sciatica. We are aware that an increase in interdiskal pressure causes pain. It is known that if traction is applied 2 weeks postsurgery to nylon sutures, which are attached to ligamentous structures, pressure on the sutures fastened to the posterior-longitudinal ligaments or the posterior aspects of the annulus fibrosis will cause pain. In addition, there are pathoanatomical studies showing that low back pain occurs clinically long before the radiological changes that follow this rupture are manifested. (For a list of references, see ref. 23.)

The incidence of back pain incapacity in industry is high and it is fair to say that it is approximately the same in all countries—around 6%. Back pain is obviously also on the march. Why it is increasing is difficult to say. Nevertheless, a consideration of industry-associated back pain leads us into the biomechanical components of the condition, and measurements have been made in our own laboratories since the fifties (24). Essentially, these experiments were designed to evaluate the effects of various positions and working tasks on the spine. At first, cadaver samples were used and they behaved hydrostatically, which simply means that it was possible to measure both the pressure and the tangential stresses in the annulus fibrosis. These stresses were very high, about four or five times that of the applied load (21). Recently, several experiments were performed in Chicago demonstrating that the pressure does not increase very much with backward bending (29). However, once total laminectomy has been performed, the pressure increases greatly, and one can demonstrate that this increase is greater with rotation and backward extension than with flexion. What this means is that if one disturbs the motion of the segment too greatly during surgery, then one creates what can be called an instability of this segment. This is a message for the surgeon to take care!

There are a variety of methods with which one may study loads in industry. We have used quantitative electromyography in particular. Computer technology can convert the electromyogram in such a way that the irregular pattern is integrated into something that can then be quantified in microvolts (3).

If one assumes that standing produces 100% load, this represents about 40 to 50 kg of load at the third lumbar disk. Bending increases this by 50% and adding 10 kg weight by 120%. Sitting unsupported increses the load by 40% because in this instance, the line of gravity falls in front of the L3 disk. A summary of the results from disk pressure studies are given in the table.

There are a few papers that demonstrate that Williams Flexion Exercises do more harm than Nature's own course of treatment. If the individual who has been off from work for a long time is to reduce the amount of load put on the back during muscle-strengthening exercises, the exercises should be performed isometrically. This will reduce the total load on the spine (27). From observations of the way people sit at work, in wheelchairs, in offices, and in automobiles, it is evident that the load on the spine can be markedly reduced by inclining the backrest and providing

TABLE 1. *Approximate load on L3-disk in a person weighing 70 kg*

Activity	N*
Supine, awake	250
Supine, semi-Fowler position	100
Supine, traction 500 N	0
Supine, tilt table 50°	400
Supine, arm exercises	500
Upright, sitting without support	700
Sitting with lumbar support backrest inclination 110°	400
Standing, at ease	500
Coughing	600
Straining	600
Forward bend 20°	600
Forward bend 40°	1000
Forward bend 20° with 20 kg	1200
Forward flexed 20° and rotated 20° with 10 kg	2100
Sitting-up exercises	1200
Bilateral leg lift	800
Lifting 10 kg, back straight	1700
Lifting 10 kg, back bent	1900
Holding 5 kg, arms extended	1900

*Newton = unit of force in SI-system. It is defined as the force necessary to give a mass of 1 kg the acceleration of 1 meter/sec^2.

1 N = 0.102 kp. For practical purposes, 10 N = 1 kp.

a lumbar support and armrests. A closer look at back pain in industry revealed an interesting fact relating to the way in which people lift objects. Although we are taught that one should lift heavy weights with the back straight and legs flexed, this method brings a much greater muscle mass into play; this, while favoring the spine, requires more work by the heart. Therefore, the "wrong way" of lifting in fact favors cardiac function.

Experimentally, a good correlation was shown between the electromyographic signal and an increasing load in the hands at various degrees of flexion. Electromyography was performed only at the L3 level. Collaborative studies with Schultz produced an excellent correlation between his models and our measurements in different positions of the spine (Schultz, A. B., Andersson, G. B. J., Örtengren, R., Haderspeck, K., and Nachemson, A.: Loads on the lumbar spine: Validation of a biomechanical analysis by measurements of intradiscal pressure and myoelectric signals. *In preparation*.) Myoelectric activity correlated well with spinal tension. Although this correlation was not perfect in all positions, its relationship with lumbar disk pressures and mean spine compression has given us for the first time the possibility of calculating—on the basis of films of patients at the worksite—how much of the load is on the disks. This also means that we now have the possibility of determining whether or not mechanical factors are of any importance at all in the production of back pain.

Diskography has been singularly unrewarding and has not yielded very much information other than to reveal some incipient disk degeneration. What may be more important, however, is the biochemical makeup of the disk. The pH within the disk is sometimes low and correlates well with the lactate concentration, which may be increased. Likewise, the PO_2 is very low—in the order of only a few mm Hg. However, most of the disk's metabolism is anaerobic. Most of the nutrients gain access to the disk through the end-plates and not via the capillaries in the annulus. Other studies have shown that solutes move by molecular diffusion whereas some macromolecules accompany fluid movements into and out of the disk. Also, we have found that anions travel via the annulus and cations via the end-plates. These studies demonstrated that vascular contacts in the bone and the subchondral bone and the cartilage of the end-plates were implicated in diffusion into the disks. Furthermore, it has been demonstrated that end-plate permeability decreases with increasing age. These findings have been corroborated by animal experiments in which active dogs were compared with inactive dogs that were confined to cages. A 15% increase in sulfur turnover was noted in the active animals. Movement might therefore be beneficial to disk nutrition.

From an analysis of the disk components, it can be demonstrated that the inner part of the annulus fibrosis is the most heavily stressed portion; this is corroborated by examination of the pathoanatomical slices which show that this is the first area to break down. Some form of degeneration occurs in between the inner lamellae, leading to separation of these structures. There are both chemical and mathematical explanations for this occurrence. The resulting separation of the lamellae thus weakens the structure of the annulus. Therefore, when the disk pressures are particularly high, the weakened annulus is then likely to give way, thereby causing the disk to rupture.

It is well recognized clinically that a disk rupture takes "forever" to heal. The turnover time of chondriotin sulfate in the nucleus pulposus is approximately 400 days in the dog and over 700 days in the human. Since these substances are necessary for the production of the glycosoaminoglycans that constitute the disk matrix, it will obviously take in excess of 2 years for the disk to heal once a rupture has occurred, unless extensive ingrowth of granulation tissue occurs from the outside.

An interesting sidelight to the space exploration programs is the finding that astronauts are prone to back pain immediately after their period of weightlessness. During weightlessness, their disks increase in size because of the inward movement of fluid, such that their overall body length increases by as much as 5 cm. Pain is felt as the disks return to their normal size. Water moves into the disks apparently because of the movement of negatively charged ions of chondroitin sulfate and keratan sulfate. Disk hydration is counterbalanced by external compression, by the annulus fibrosis, and by internal collagen fiber tension. This increased hydration alters the mechanical properties of the disk, at least the intradiskal pressure, and this in turn increases the stress on the posterior part of the annulus. Disk hydration and increased size also occur, to a lesser degree, during sleep, and therefore, we should warn our patients, "Be careful in the morning."

Pain fibers have been demonstrated in the outer part of the annulus fibrosis. None are found within the disks. Pain transmitted by these fibers can be referred to the nerve that supplies the facetal joints and to the superficial muscles and skin.

We are also aware that pain mechansms can be altered not only at the source of nociception but also by modulation in the dorsal root entry zone. Pain arising in one segment can be amplified in another segment, and because it can cross over to the other side of the cord via internuncial connections, it can cross over to the other side of the body. This explains why procedures like chordotomy are rarely successful.

The burgeoning information relating to the endorphins includes some interesting features. Patients with chronic back pain have lower cerebrospinal fluid levels of these peptides than normal people, thus raising the possibility of a pharmacological approach to the alleviation of their symptoms. In addition, it has been shown that transcutaneous nerve stimulation and acupuncture also increase the production of endorphins, which probably explains in part the success of these forms of treatment in certain pain states, including low back pain.

Whereas most of the foregoing discussion is of a descriptive nature where I have attempted to catalog the features and etiology of back pain, the remaining section will deal more with the prevention of low back pain. Is prevention possible? The answer to this question is not clear. Until recently, it was not possible to apply successful preventive measures because the information relating to mechanical factors and also psychological and sociological factors was not known. Without this information, it was not possible to initiate any form of program that could be used in elementary school, and it is there that the teaching of posture and the importance of its relationship to subsequent back pathology should be initiated. The next resort is to introduce such knowledge during vocational education. Finally, it is at the work site that most attention must be paid, and the application of ergonomics, as the science of obtaining the best fit between the machine and the worker, must follow.

Secondary prevention includes the advice that one gives to patients regarding their everyday activities. This especially includes work, and each one of us should be in a position to inform our patients before they go back to work that there are certain positions and tasks that must be avoided. These are measurable quantities. Patients should avoid twisting, heavy lifting, and sitting without arm and lumbar support. Also, as has been mentioned above, maintaining physical fitness through exercise increases the delivery of nutrients to the disks and increases the cerebrospinal fluid content of endorphins. It is now well known that certain exercises such as walking, jogging, bicycling, swimming, and cross-country skiing are definitely less taxing to the back than other forms of exercise.

Now let us consider a rational approach to the management of back pain. A constant difficulty associated with management is the failure to separate acute from chronic back pain. The treatment of low back pain is certainly not synonymous with the treatment of sciatica. Sciatica results from a disk herniation that is generally well managed and responds to appropriate therapy. The treatment of acute low back pain has also produced positive results in prospectively well-controlled series. Rothman and his co-workers showed recently that a combination of bed rest and salicylates is highly successful for acute low back pain, but the effects of this treatment should not be extrapolated to the long-term sufferer. In fact, a program initiated in Gothenborg during 1965 was designed to provide an educational experience and create confidence in the patients by avoiding excessive therapy (40). The patients were taught to lie in the semi-Fowler position in order to deload the spine. Following initial instruction on the nature of their condition, the patients then undertook their second lesson when they were taught some low-pressure resting positions and exercises. If muscular training was needed for this stage, isometrics were taught. The third lesson, which is the most important, was ergonomics and its practical application to future activity. Finally, the physical therapists who worked with the patients accompanied them to their worksite where the practical application of the rehabilitation period was undertaken.

A 5-year study using the foregoing principles was undertaken by an orthopedic resident and a physical therapist with the workers at the Volvo Company in Sweden (7). Patients were selected for the study on the basis of an acute episode of low back pain, providing there was no prior history of such pain. The study involved 210 subjects who were randomly allocated to the Back School or to a conventional physiotherapy program, which contained a number of modalities including manipulation, and to a placebo group. During the first year of the study, each subject was assessed by an orthopedic surgeon no less than five times. The follow-up included every subject, that is, 100% of the subjects.

The results were as follows: First, following initial treatment, the duration of pain in the Back School and physical therapy patient groups was 15 days less than that in the placebo group—a significant difference. The obvious conclusion from this was that taking care of the patient helped to bring about a more rapid resolution of symptoms. Second, there was a significant difference between the two first groups regarding their ability to return to work: the Back School patients returned 1 week sooner. These findings indicate that advice based on knowledge is better than treatment based on armchair pathology!

What about the treatment of chronic back pain patients? Williams flexion and muscle-strengthening exercises, which are used so universally in conjunction with shortwave and ultrasound therapy, have never been shown to produce any great benefit for patients with chronic back pain. Back manipulation has been shown to be similarly ineffective. There are approximately 20 prospectively controlled studies of various types of manipulations. These procedures seem to help males with acute symptoms for an hour or two, but they do not diminish the overall sickness period (10,34).

Both anti-inflammatory drugs and injection therapy have proved to be failures. The use of corsets to splint the back have met with mixed results, probably because we are still lacking any good prospective trials. Traction, facet injections, and comprehensive back care programs are now blossoming in the United States. The results of these programs are still not yet available and, therefore, it is not possible to comment on them. However, there are reports demonstrating that it is nearly impossible to rehabilitate patients with chronic low back pain after they have been off from work for a year or more (1).

Acute sciatica is a condition in which there have been good prospective studies that demonstrate beneficial results from epidural steroid injection. Autotraction, introduced by Lind, has produced some remarkable results. We studied 82 patients between the ages of 20 and 55, all of whom had markedly reduced straight-leg raising because of their radiculopathy. They were allocated into two treatment groups. One group was treated with the usual pain-killing pills and/or a corset, and the other group received autotraction. The average number of autotraction sessions was 2.5. Results were as follows: After 1 week, 17 of the autotraction patients were greatly improved whereas only two in the corset group showed any improvement. After 3 weeks, and even more after 3 months, these differences diminished because natural resolution entered into the results, but the fact remains that those in the autotraction group showed a statistically significant short-term improvement in their condition without any diminution of the improvement over the longer period.

What is the role of surgery? Certainly, if a herniated disk is found, it should be removed. Under these circumstances, one can obtain almost a 100% relief of sciatica. If there is incomplete herniation or just a bulging disk without any herniation, the results of surgery are worse than no treatment at all, worse than the natural history of the condition. The use of metrizamide is discussed by David Berg elsewhere in this volume, and it serves as a good example of a means of positively identifying the presence of a disk herniation. It is imperative that the identification be made before any surgery is contemplated. Another consideration is that the symptoms should not be more than 4 to 5 months old because the longer these symptoms are present, the sooner the behavioral aspects of chronic pain begin to manifest themselves. It is much better to have surgery before any deep psychological disturbances are manifested. The technique is not to remove too much; then results yielding better than 90% of relief of symptoms can be obtained for the leg pain. Patients should be told, however, that their back pain might still prevail.

Chymopapain has enjoyed a limited success. However, no prospective controlled studies have been done. The technique is presently again under review in a triple-blind multi-center study now being performed in the United States (see Wilkinson, *this volume*).

For chronic sciatica, there have been no positive results in any controlled series, so what options are available? One can perform spinal fusion, or undertake facet injection and/or denervation of the facetal joint. In one relatively well-controlled series that included only 40 patients, it was shown that facet injection seemed to provide some statistically significant improvement. Epidural steroid injection is also being used, but again it is not clear what percentage of patients are benefited by this procedure.

Spinal stenosis is another condition that may be amenable to surgery, particularly in those who have symptoms mimicking intermittent claudication. Before surgery is considered, both radiographic and myelographic changes should be present. The type of pain is unique and tends to increase during the day, particularly with downhill walking, compared with other forms of back pain due to mechanical defects, which typically increases with uphill walking. Obviously, pain of vascular origin must be excluded. The most important thing in this diagnosis is positive-contrast myelography that demonstrates a dural sac of less than 10 mm in diameter.

A related disorder that is of particular concern to physicians in the United States is root canal stenosis that causes nerve entrapment. It is not really known how often this occurs and at which point it becomes the genesis of pain. We do not know how to avoid the scarring that occurs after surgery, and again, there are no prospective controlled studies in this area. However, one thing that is certain is that once a total laminectomy has been performed, the motion segment is weakened; spinal fusion is then necessary, at least when the patient is fairly young.

Instability of the motion segment is a rather vague description. I would consider the condition present when X-rays show about 4 mm of translatory motion on bending and more than 15° angulation between the vertebral bodies (25).

As mentioned above, surgery for true disk herniation can achieve only 40 to 50% relief of back pain; moreover, the etiology of back pain in this condition is still unknown. Another factor associated with surgery is a 4 to 5% recurrence rate requiring further surgery either at the same or at another level. There are very poor data on the results of repeated surgery, and in the best of hands, only 30% of patients are improved after the second operation, and only 5% of those undergoing surgery a fourth time obtain relief (36). Thus, it would appear that an axiom for disk surgery is that there is only one chance of curing the patient. We must also keep in mind the natural history of disk disease, that is, in the majority of cases, if one waits long enough, the disease is self-limiting or unchangeable by surgical intervention.

We also previously discussed background factors such as the work situation, the patient's social situation, and psychological makeup. In two separate studies of 200 patients each, Wadell looked for nonorganic signs that should be sought before one considered reoperating on patients with low back pain (36). He found that certain psychological stigmata correlated well with the reoperative rate. Six tests were performed to elucidate the psychological makeup. The first simulates what the patient thinks is a load on his spine by placing one's hands on the patient's head. In the second test, the patient's body is swung to the left and right such that the main motion occurs at the knees and hip joint rather than at the spine. A positive test consists of the patient reacting with strong pain. Thirdly, the back is palpated for extensive nonorganic tenderness. Fourthly, areas of stocking anesthesia in the lower limbs are sought. Fifthly, a false-positive straight-leg raising is sought. Finally, if there is an overreaction to examination and if five out of these six tests give positive results, surgery should not be performed.

In summary, we discussed both primary and secondary prevention and also what might correctly be considered tertiary prevention, that is, preventing surgery because this modality is still one of the most important factors for creating chronic back cripples. We have to look at the whole picture and we certainly have to determine a better means of treatment than we presently have.

Better prospective controlled studies are needed, studies that do not mix apples with oranges, chronic low back pain patients with those who have acute sciatica. Better use of existing knowledge of psychosocial, ergonomical, mechanical, chemical, and neurophysiological factors will also help to solve some of the problems of this very complicated and presently frustrating condition—low back pain.

REFERENCES

1. Åberg, J. (1980): Hur framgångsrik är Ryggrehabilitering. Utvärdering av verksamheten vid Rygginstitutet i Sundsvall. Socialmedicinsk tidskrifts skriftserie, nr 44.
2. Andersson, G., Örtengren, R., and Nachemson, A. (1976): Quantitative studies of back loads in lifting. *Spine*, 1:178–185.
3. Andersson, G., Örtengren, R., and Nachemson, A. (1977): Intradiskal pressure, intra-abdominal pressure and myoelectric back muscle activity related to posture and loading. *Clin. Orthop.*, 129:156–164.
4. Andersson, G., Örtengren, R., and Nachemson, A. (1978): Quantitative studies of the load on the back in different working postures. *Scand. J. Rehabil. Med.*, *(Suppl.)* 6:173–181.
5. Andersson, G., Örtengren, R., Nachemson, A., and Elfström, G. (1974): Lumbar disc pressure and myoelectric back muscle activity during sitting. IV. Studies on a car driver's seat. *Scand. J. Rehabil. Med.*, 6:128–133.
6. Andersson, G., and Schultz, A. B. (1979): Effects of fluid injections on mechanical properties of intervertebral discs. *J. Biomech.*, 12:453–458.
7. Bergquist-Ullman, M., and Larsson, U. (1977): Acute low back pain in industry. A controlled prospective study with special reference to therapy and confounding factors. *Acta Orthop. Scand. (Suppl.)*, 170.
8. Davis, P. R. (1972): The physical causation of disease. *R. Soc. Health J.*, 92:63–64.
9. Diamant, B., Karlsson, J., and Nachemson, A. (1978): Correlation between lactate levels and pH in discs of patients with lumbar rhizopathies. *Experientia*, 24:1195–1196.
10. Glover, J. R., Morris, J. G., and Khosla, T. (1974): Back pain: A randomized clinical trial of rotational manipulation of the trunk. *Br. J. Ind. Med.*, 31:59–64.
11. Hansson, T. (1977): The bone mineral content and biomechanical properties of lumbar vertebrae. An in vitro study based on dual photon absorptiometry. University of Göteborg, thesis.
12. Holm, S. (1980): Nutrition of the intervertebral disc. Transport and metabolism. University of Göteborg, thesis.
13. Horal, J. (1969): The clinical appearance of low back disorders in the city of Gothenburg, Sweden. *Acta Orthop. Scand. (Suppl.)*, 118.
14. Kelsey, J. L., and White, A. A. (1980): Epidemiology and impact of low-back pain. *Spine*, 5:133–142.
15. Larsson, U., Chöler, U., Lidström, A., Lind, G., Nachemson, A., Nilsson, B., and Roslund, J. (1980): Auto-traction for treatment of lumbago–sciatica. *Acta Orthop. Scand.*, 51:791–799.
16. Lewin, T. (1964): Osteoarthritis in lumbar synovial joints. A morphologic study. The Department of Anatomy and the Department of Orthopaedics, Gothenburg, Sweden, thesis.
17. Lidström, A., and Zachrisson, M. (1970): Physical therapy on low back pain and sciatica. *Scand. J. Rehabil. Med.*, 2:37–42.
18. Lind, G. A. M. (1974): Auto-traction. Treatment of low back pain and sciatica. *Linköpings University*, *Medical Dissertations*, No. 17, the Regional Hospital, Linköping, Sweden, thesis.
19. Magora, A., and Schwartz, A. (1968): Relation between low back pain and x-ray changes. 4. Lysis and olisthesis. *Scand. J. Rehabil. Med.*, 12:47–52.

20. Maroudas, A., Stockwell, R. A., Nachemson, A., and Urban, J. P. G. (1975): Factors involved in the nutrition of the human lumbar intervertebral disc: cellularity and diffusion of glucose in vitro. *J. Anat.*, 120, 1:113–130.
21. Nachemson, A. (1965): The load on lumbar disks in different positions of the body. *Clin. Orthop.*, 45:107–122.
22. Nachemson, A. (1975): Towards a better understanding of low back pain. A review of the mechanics of the lumbar disc. *Rheumatol. Rehabil.*, 14:129–143.
23. Nachemson, A. (1976): The lumbar spine. An orthopaedic challenge. *Spine*, 1:59–71.
24. Nachemson, A. (1980): Lumbar intradiscal pressure. In: *The Lumbar Spine and Back Pain*, 2nd ed., edited by M. Jayson, pp. 341–358. Pitman Medical Publishing Co., Ltd., Turnbridgewells, Kent, United Kingdom.
25. Nachemson, A. (1981): Instability—diagnostic criterions. *Spine*, *(in press)*.
26. Nachemson, A. (1981): Disc pressure measurements. *Spine*, 6:93–97.
27. Nachemson, A., and Elfström, G. (1970): Intravital dynamic pressure measurements in lumbar discs. A study of common movements, maneuvres and exercises. *Scand. J. Rehabil. Med.*, *(Suppl.)*, 1:1–40.
28. Nachemson, A., Lewin, T., Maroudas, A., and Freeman, M. A. R. (1970): In vitro diffusion of dye through the end-plates and the annulus fibrosus of human lumbar intervertebral discs. *Acta Orthop. Scand.*, 41:589–607.
29. Nachemson, A., Schultz, A. B., and Berkson, M. H. (1979): Mechanical properties of human lumbar spine motion segments. Influences of age, sex, disc level and degeneration. *Spine*, 4:1–8.
30. Porter, R. W., Hibbert, C. S., and Wicks, M. (1978): The spinal canal in symptomatic lumbar disc lesions. *J. Bone Joint Surg.*, 60B:4:485.
31. Ramani, P. S., Perry, R. H., and Tomlinson, B. E. (1975): Role of ligamentum flavum in the symptomatology of prolapsed lumbar intervertebral discs. *J. Neurol. Neurosurg. Psychiatry*, 38:550–557.
32. Schultz, A. B., Warwick, D. N., Berkson, M. H., and Nachemson, A. (1979): Mechanical properties of human lumbar spine motion segments. Part I: Responses in flexion, extension, lateral bending and torsion. *J. Biomech. Eng.*, 101:46–52.
33. Shealy, C. N. (1974): The role of the spinal facets in back and sciatic pain. *Headache*, 14:101–104.
34. Sims-Williams, H., Jayson, M. I. V., Young, S. M. S., Badderley, H., and Collins, E. (1978): Controlled trial of mobilization and manipulation for patients with low back pain in general practice. *Brit. Med. J.*, 2:1338–1340.
35. Urban, J. P. G., Holm, S., Maroudas, A., and Nachemson, A. (1977): Nutrition of the intervertebral disk. An in vivo study of solute transport. *J. Clin. Orthop.*, 129:101–114.
36. Waddell, G., McCulloch, J. A., Kummel, E., and Venner, R. M. (1980): Nonorganic physical signs in low back pain. *Spine*, 5:117–125.
37. Weber, H. (1978): Lumbar disc herniation. A prospective study of prognostic factors including a controlled trial. Neurological Department, Ullevål Hospital, Oslo, Norway, thesis.
38. Westrin, C.-G. (1973): Low back sick-listing. A nosological and medical insurance investigation. *Scand. J. Soc. Med.*, *(Suppl.)*, 7:1–116.
39. Wood, P. H. N., and Badley, E. M. (1980): Epidemiology of back pain. In: *The Lumbar Spine and Back Pain*, 2nd ed., edited by M. Jayson, pp. 29–55. Pitman Medical Publishing Co. Ltd., Tunbridge Wells, Kent, United Kingdom.
40. Zachrisson, M. (1981): The back school. *Spine*, 6:104–106.

Chronic Low Back Pain, edited by
M. Stanton-Hicks and Robert Boas.
Raven Press, New York © 1982.

Assessment and Management Planning of Chronic Low Back Pain

P. Prithvi Raj, James E. McLennan, and James C. Phero

Pain Control Center, University of Cincinnati Medical Center, Cincinnati, Ohio 45267

The genre of chronic low back and lower extremity pain lends itself to a scenario that involves the inception and evolution of physiologic and behavioral changes, clearly separating this entity from its acute counterpart. Clinical evaluation and therapy within the setting of a multidisciplinary pain control center are currently the most fruitful mechanisms to achieve at least partial reversal of chronic changes, which have usually been reinforced by a number of different physicians and modalities of treatment. It is essential to realize at the outset that patients who reach a stage of chronicity (defined as 3 to 6 months of continuous pain) may no longer be viewed or treated in terms of the two major acute syndromes of low back and leg pain commonly presenting to physicians, namely, lumbosacral nerve root compression with referred pain in the appropriate dermatome and acute low back "strain" with ligamentous and muscle compromise. Although both these situations apply in the chronic state as well, the solutions in the latter are considerably more difficult than the classic therapy of relieving root pressure (e.g., surgical disk excision or heat, rest, and pharmacologic therapy for muscle spasm).

The patient presenting at a multidisciplinary pain center for diagnosis and treatment of chronic low back pain has generally been failed by the ministrations of several physicians. It is noteworthy here that the published results of surgical therapy of acute low back radicular syndromes are probably more encouraging than the careful analysis of long-term results would substantiate (16). Even with entirely appropriate initial therapy, a chronic pain state may evolve and be compounded by repeated operations. Depending on a patient's initial cultural, social, and economic background attitudes, he has usually proceeded through a "pain scenario" (Fig. 1) involving anatomic and physiologic manipulations; these additionally injure the involved tissues, initiate reflex mechanisms to intensify pain in regional or distant tissues, and often serve to reinforce the patient's belief that he has a serious problem. Pain behavior develops during this period of reinforcement, further reinforced by such complicating factors as drug dependence and financial and psychologic secondary gain and compensation.

"Trauma" involving the low back that occurs while the individual is employed by another person or on the premises of an employing company is closely linked to the complex secondary gain situation and may thus have serious ramifications

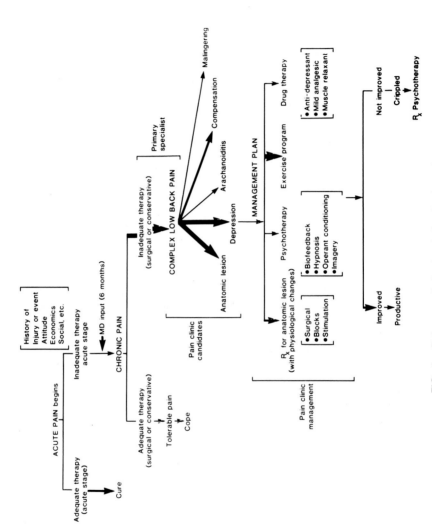

FIG. 1. Pain scenario in chronic low back syndrome.

with peers, family members, the medical community, and state and federal agencies (17). The idea that "someone is to blame for my predicament" justifies prolonged battles over compensation for injury, suffering, and loss of income. In many patients with low back pain, failure to deal explicitly with the secondary gain factor and to recognize the psychosomatic component of the problem leads to futile attempts to alleviate the patients' suffering (18,55,56).

Case History: E. M.

A 39-year-old mother of two teenage girls presented to one of the authors (J. E. McLennan) with chronic low back pain of 2 years' duration. She had originally injured her back while lifting cases of beer and was admitted to the hospital the morning after injury for myelography and 3 weeks of bed rest. Three more hospital admissions followed in the next year; her interim therapy was bed rest, a low back brace, and physical therapy. One year after injury, she underwent lumbar laminectomy and excision of the L_{4-5} disk from the left side. She remained with numbness of the lateral left foot and ankle but was free of pain until she returned to work 3 months later and was involved in a minor automobile accident.

When first seen by our group, she complained of having constant pain since the postoperative recurrence, with a periodic sharp component. Pain involved the low back and left leg. The patient's weight was 220 lb, roughly 90 lb overweight. There had been a continuing battle with workman's compensation, and she was increasingly depressed.

Physical examination showed tenderness to palpation across the lumbosacral junction and difficulty with forward and lateral bending. Epicritical cutaneous sensation was depressed in the left L_5 and S_1 dermatomes, and the left Achilles tendon response was depressed. Strength in the lower extremities was normal. Electromyography showed normal responses in all muscles of the left lower extremity; $1+$ fibrillations and positive waves were noted in the left L_5 and S_1 paraspinal muscles. The left H-reflex latency was within normal limits.

Five months later, the EMG showed marked muscle membrane instability in the paraspinal muscles of both sides, and the patient had chronic neuropathic changes in the left extensor hallucis longus. The H-reflex was now significantly prolonged on the left. Conduction velocity of the left peroneal nerve was normal. Thus, chronic recent L_5 and S_1 radiculopathy appeared to be present on the left and S_1 on the right. At this point, the patient had some early ankle weakness, particularly in dorsiflexion, and her pain had assumed a constant burning quality over much of the lower extremity on the left.

Plain lumbosacral roentgenograms were normal; there was considerable retained Pantopaque that did not move with postural changes (Fig. 2). An additional 3 ml of Pantopaque that was introduced into the subarachnoid space gave little information because scarring prevented filling of the distal thecal sac. There was diffuse narrowing and irregularity of the sac from L_4 through S_1.

Initial diagnostic root blocks were performed at L_5 and S_1 on the left with 5 ml of a solution containing 2% lidocaine and 5 mg Depo-medrol. The patient experienced rapid pain relief that lasted for approximately 4 hr, with increased sensory loss in the appropriate dermatomes. An extensive trial of four-electrode transcutaneous nerve stimulation (T.E.N.S.) was unsuccessful. Epidural instillation of 40 mg of Depo-medrol was of no benefit. Her pain rapidly worsened in the hospital. The patient maintained an active relationship with our clinical pain psychologist

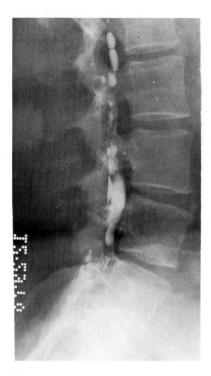 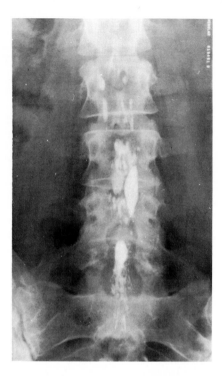

FIG. 2. In plain films of the spine (AP and lateral), Pantopaque is retained in the lumbosacral area; bony structure and interspaces are normal.

that has persisted to the current time; initial efforts were directed at relaxation imagery training and antidepressive measures.

It was decided to attempt one further surgical procedure because of the clinical and electrical evidence of progressive recent radiculopathy involving more than the originally injured root, the limited initial decompression, and the success of root blocks. She had a bilateral total lumbosacral decompression of L_5 and S_1 with exploration of the four root canals. The left L_5 root was particularly compressed by epidural scarring, and that condition was relieved. The dura was not opened. The patient was clinically much improved within a few days and began a physical therapy program that she had previously been unable to tolerate. She was sent home 2 weeks after surgery. Generally, she did well for approximately 1 year but had several setbacks related to various falls. Her self-esteem sagged severely despite continuous psychologic support; social problems were major, particularly those involving her teenage daughters and difficulties with obtaining financial support from the state workman's compensation board. During the later portion of the postoperative year, her syndrome changed. There was recurrence of the leg pain accompanied by increased ankle weakness to the point where she began using a cane and finally crutches. The motor loss was unpredictable and was related to her falls. She was unable to sit because of a burning dysesthetic sensation over the sacrum that was exacerbated by pressure. The burning sensation was present in much of the left lower extremity as well. Her EMG remained unchanged.

Succeeding therapeutic maneuvers included a series of caudal injections of local anesthetic and steroids and several sets of myoneural blocks of the gluteal and low paraspinal muscles. The patient suffered from painful muscle spasms of the buttocks and left thigh. T.E.N.S. was again unsuccessful, perhaps because of the patient's increasing obesity. Repeated myelography was undertaken, this time with metrizamide (Fig. 3); this showed little change in the conformation of the thecal sac.

Ultimately, the patient was given an implanted epidural electrode system attached to a subcutaneous receiver; this was activated by a standard external radiofrequency transmitter (Medtronics, Minneapolis, Minnesota). Electrodes were introduced at L_1 and the tips placed at T_9 and T_{10} with one anterior to the cord and one posterior (Fig. 4). Within a week, this system afforded her 85% overall relief and continues to do so presently.

ASSESSMENT

The case history traces the course of a patient with low back pain at various stages of her condition. These stages obviously do not occur in all patients, but progression of one pain syndrome to the other is common in such patients. It is for this reason that a thorough assessment is necessary. Therapeutic options are dependent on the correct diagnosis of such syndromes. Although the history of the patient's course prior to multidisciplinary evaluation is valuable, the pain center must essentially begin anew, with the *current* anatomic, physiologic, and psychologic status. All phases of the work-up should ideally proceed in parallel. After the initial visit, it is often helpful to admit the patient to the hospital for a week or so of intense documentation of the current status and perhaps initial therapy. It must be admitted that the anatomic etiology of the patient's pain may not always be clearly separated from its physiologic and psychologic components by physical, electrophysiologic, or roentgenographic examination alone. Various "tricks" must often be used to isolate the apparent anatomic pain pathway from the patient's response to pain or the anticipation thereof. "Pain memory" and cultural attitudes are critical in this regard (28,43,60). Ultimately, even maneuvers involving selective "blocking" of regional structures with local anesthetics or sham injections may not be reliable. Pain must be considered valid if the patient "suffers"; unfortunately, physical pain is only a small portion of the vast spectrum of suffering (35). The various investigative blocks, however, may furnish important clues to the management of such patients.

History

The essential points of the history are (a) the events of onset of the problem and its initial presentation, (b) evaluation of the pain characteristics to the time of multidisciplinary contact, and (c) the various interventions (surgical and otherwise) that have been made and their immediate effect on the evolution of the patient's chronic syndrome. It is generally not helpful to sort through the hundreds of radiographs accompanying many new patients or the myriad of details often recorded compulsively in a "log book"; the latter, however, is likely to amplify certain

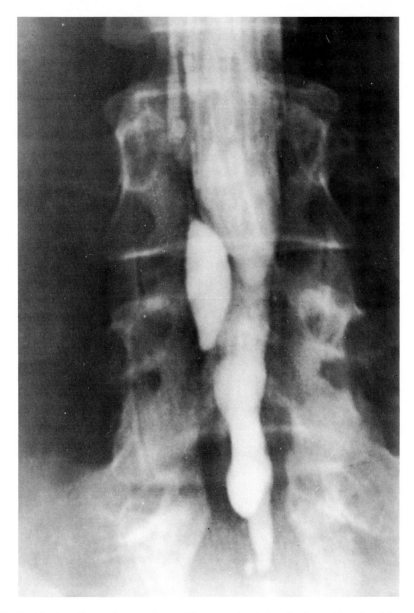

FIG. 3. Metrizamide myelogram shows diffuse scarring in the distal sac. Note the defects of loculated retained Pantopaque from the previous study.

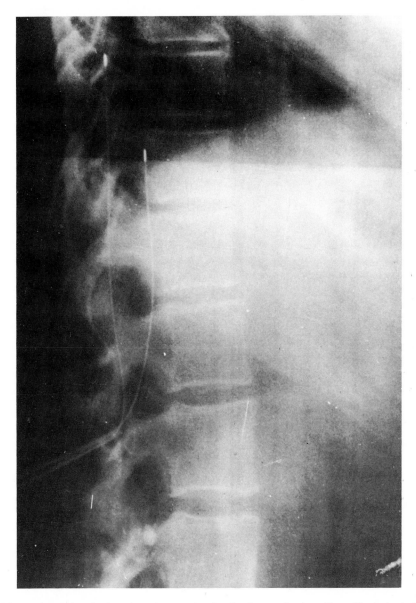

FIG. 4. Lateral projection of myelogram showing the thoraco-lumbar spine with electrode tips placed at T_9 and T_{11}.

opinions the physician is generating about the particular difficulties of achieving success in treating such a patient.

Physical Examination

What is the current status of the patient at examination? An evaluation includes (a) low back and lower extremity anatomy, (b) likely tissues of origin for the pain and physiologic changes due to chronicity, and (c) functional assessment of physical and psychologic capabilities. If the patient's life style is minimally altered, except for the absence of gainful employment, and the physical examination is essentially unremarkable, little can be accomplished in reversing the patient's behavior pattern. It is essential to triage patients after the initial workup, so that efforts are not expended on a defined group of poor responders.

In an attempt to define which structures hurt and why they hurt, the physical evaluation begins with the patient's description of the site, temporal patterns, and varying intensities of pain. The patient's perception of pain may have little to do with the structures actually producing or modifying it. Immediately, one is involved with the "language of pain"; mutual interpretation by physician and patient of adjectives describing pain are the basis for the initial diagnosis as to its etiology and mechanism (33,46).

Physical examination should include evaluating the essentials of the patient's systemic status: obvious respiratory or cardiac problems and signs and symptoms of diffuse disease involving joints, muscles, or the neurologic system, which must involve other specialists. In focusing on chronic low back pain, evaluation is made of skeletal, myofascial, and nervous system anatomy and function. Obviously, normal nervous system function may transmit to consciousness pain from aberrant function of the musculoskeletal system.

Skeletal Evaluation

The patient should be entirely disrobed. Curvature of the spinal axis should be noted. The presence of reduced or exaggerated lordosis or of kyphosis or scoliosis indicates muscle imbalance usually from spasm, weakness or bony abnormality. Most scoliosis, on its own merit, is not painful. Is the abnormal curvature fixed? Is the range of motion of the spine abnormal and accompanied by increased symptomatology? Is there traumatic vertebral joint movement limitation or surgical fusion? Can pain be attributed to a "facet syndrome"? Has the patient had prior myelography, laminectomy, and disk excision or fusion? Are appropriate scars present? Is there evidence of congenital or progressive spinal deformity, e.g., spondylosis, spondylolysis, spondylolisthesis, spina bifida occulta, etc.?

Range of motion of the hips, knees, and ankles should be studied in relation to pain production. Is there joint disease or other orthopedic deformity, chronic sepsis of bone or joints, osteoporosis, etc.? Pain may be initiated by any of these structures and actually attributed to nerve roots or more proximal structures. One must not focus only on the low back and attribute lower level pain to known pathways of peripheral distribution of roots without thoroughly evaluating the distal structures themselves.

Vigorous percussion and palpation is made along the spinous processes in order to search for focal tenderness or trigger points leading to radiation of pain. The gait is often extremely revealing, particularly if observed without the patient's knowledge. Many patients use support devices, e.g., canes, crutches, braces, corsets, etc., which are often improperly fitted and used.

Neuromuscular Evaluation

The entire musculature of the back and the lower extremities should be examined. Frequently, a remote fasciculation may be noted while attention is focused on another area of the body. Muscle bulk, atrophy, and symmetry should be evaluated. Measurements comparing the two sides may aid in identifying subtle differences. Are there tender muscle bellies or insertions? Palpation of the muscles in relation to the course of the sciatic nerve is made from the sciatic notch to mid-calf. Is the nerve tender or enlarged? Atrophy may be due to lower motor neuron lesions or to disuse from chronic upper motor neuron loss or pain. Is focal paralysis or weakness present? Are fasciculations visible? Do they follow the distribution of a single root indicating chronic irritation? It should be determined if the distribution of weakness comes from one or more roots, a peripheral nerve, or primary muscle disease. Are there distal changes in the lower extremity indicating peripheral neuropathy? These generally involve both motor and sensory patterns and present with other confirmatory findings in the neurologic examination. If weakness is discovered, it is important to know whether or not there has been progression to other muscle groups and to quantify the weakness. Is loss of function accompanied by a flaccid state, as is the usual case in lesions peripheral to the spinal cord, or by spasticity? It is essential to have the patient's cooperation in testing muscle strength. Often observation is more reliable in terms of functional impairment. Many patients with low back pain tolerance or with hysteria will not hold a muscle against resistance; this presents as a sudden "give out" during examination. Generally, if the muscle can even briefly be contracted fully, it is normal. The patient's weight may be used to evaluate lower extremity strength by having the patient stand on the toes and heels.

Deep Tendon Reflexes

Deep tendon reflexes (DTRs) test the monosynaptic reflex pathways from muscle stretch receptors through the lower spinal cord and back to the effector response in the muscle of origin. Suppression indicates lower motor-neuron interruption, and exaggeration usually results from a "release" phenomenon of lesions at the cord or higher in the nervous system. Symmetry is important, particularly at the ankles where the Achilles tendon response is frequently depressed bilaterally in older patients. The monosynaptic "H" reflex measures a similar pathway electrically in the sciatic nerve.

Although multiple nerve root involvement is common in patients with chronic low back disease, one should not overlook the possibility of intraspinal or lumbar plexus tumor in this condition. The pattern of loss should be fairly constant in benign disease and progressive in the case of tumor. Most patients with chronic depression of reflexes will retain this loss despite alleviation of their symptoms.

Cutaneous Sensation

An attempt should be made to define a pattern of loss in the sensory examination. Sensory loss is very subjective and often misleading or inconsistent on subsequent examinations, particularly if multiple root distributions are involved. Persistence of sensory loss from prior resolved syndromes is common. Do the sensory and motor findings indicate the same distribution of loss? Superficial cutaneous reflexes, such as the cremasteric and abdominal responses, are not of much value in confirming the presence of focal disease.

Determining the Source of Pain

Pain Originating in Myofascial Tissue

Palpation is made to discover areas of muscle that cause focal or radiating pain. These may be "trigger zones" or tight bands of muscle fibers leading to a "jump sign" (53,59). The complex of myofascial syndromes has been discussed for over 50 years and is still poorly understood. Nonetheless, it is frequently a major portion of the patient's disability (23). A common syndrome involves progression of pain from paraspinal muscles to the muscles attached to the iliac crest; these in turn cause tension at the greater tuberosity and produce tenderness of the iliotibial tract. These myofascial syndromes may mimic those caused by nerve root lesions (Fig. 5).

Pain Originating in Nerve Tissue

Classically, one finds severe, acute, radiating pain on movement. This may be caused by nerve root entrapment at the intervertebral foramina or compression in the spinal canal. The straight-leg raising, for example, stretches the sciatic nerve and transmits tension to the plexus and roots of L_4, L_5, and S_1. An important differential point is the separation of sciatic irritation by this mechanism from that caused by the recently identified mechanism, a narrow lumbar spinal canal (31,34,61). In the latter condition, the patient may also complain of pain along the distribution of the sciatic nerve, exaggerated by walking and often involving both lower extremities. The sciatic stretch test is negative. The patient has pain on hyperextension of the spine rather than flexion; the hypertrophic ligamentum flavum buckles during hyperextension and compresses the roots of the cauda equina between itself and the anterior canal margin. Patients with narrow spinal canal syndromes will often be most comfortable lying on the abdomen with thighs flexed or walking in kyphosis

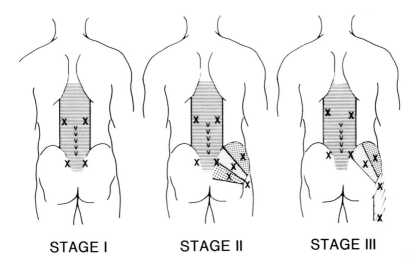

STAGE I   STAGE II   STAGE III

FIG. 5. Common areas of pain and muscle spasm in myofascial pain syndromes. **Stage I** = Bilateral paravertebral muscle spasm and tenderness. **Stage II** = Paravertebral muscles and gluteal muscles involved. Involvement of pyriformis muscle may produce sciatica. **Stage III** = Paravertebral and gluteal muscles and iliotibial tract involved. **X** = trigger point.

and in truncal flexion. Diagnosis is difficult without myelography or lumbar tommography. Lateral bending of the spine may pinch ipsilateral roots if they have insufficient space at the root canal or if intraspinal contents are bulky. Patients with severe sciatica modify their gait to avoid stretching the nerve. If a narrow lumbar canal is suspected, it is vital to assess the status of the peripheral circulation in the lower extremities to differentiate neurogenic claudication from true arterial claudication. Fixed nerve root pain may be present in vascular and infectious radiculopathies.

Visceral-Somatic Pain

Pain, tenderness, and muscle spasm in the low back may also be due to visceral pathology. In women, malposition of the uterus, endocervicitis, dysmenorrhea, salpingitis, and pelvic tumors can cause low back pain. However, it must be emphasized that most cases of backache in women are not of visceral origin but are musculoskeletal in nature and caused by ligamentous strain or nerve entrapment (13). Urethritis in women, disease of the prostate and posterior urethra in men, and ureteral calculi in both sexes can cause backaches. The importance of a pelvic and rectal examination is thus obvious.

Pain in the low back syndrome may, by this stage in the examination, be roughly categorized into (a) neurogenic, (b) myofascial, (c) skeletal, and (d) visceral–somatic. If it fits none of these categories, further investigations are necessary to determine the pain caused by reflex causalgic or psychogenic mechanisms.

There is a frequent overlap or coexistence of more than one of the above categories of pain etiology; the initial pure injury evolves to a state of chronic maintenance by spread to regional tissues and is accompanied by psychogenic responses of the patient and behavioral changes, which further modify the original pain. Thus, a patient presenting with a "simple" disk protrusion who has had appropriate surgical therapy may, if pain persists in a single root distribution, ultimately arrive at a state of diffuse tenderness of the paraspinal and gluteal muscles and iliotibial tract with chronic disuse atrophy of the involved leg. The patient views himself as an invalid, with major consequences on life style and economic status that compound the problem for his family. In this sense, the spectrum of chronic back pain cannot be overemphasized.

Investigative Procedures

Radiographic Evaluation

This is made to support the clinical impression or furnish additional information. Plain films of the lumbosacral spine should be made in the AP, lateral, and oblique views. In patients with chronic back pain, common findings are diffuse osteoarthritis with hypertrophy of the facet joints, multiple disk space collapse, and autofusion with anterior and posterior "bony bridging" across the interspaces. Are congenital anomalies present, such as defects in the pars interarticularis with spondylolisthesis, transitional vertebrae, etc.? As mentioned above, the canal diameter cannot be adequately evaluated on plain films. Tomography is important for this and also to discover details of old healed fractures or fusion competency. Flexion/extension views give information about abnormal mobility of the lumbar joints.

Films should also be made of the hips and lower extremities as the need arises. Changes from chronic disuse of an extremity will ultimately involve bone and may be the cause of chronic pain, although the original lesion is more proximal.

Myelography

Most patients with chronic back pain have experienced repeated myelography (15). This is unfortunate since the test itself may contribute to the disability. At best, it is a transiently irritating procedure; at its extreme, it may cause progressive arachnoiditis. The newer water-soluble contrast agents, particularly metrizamide, are probably preferable in their anatomic resolution to the classic oily contrast agents like Pantopaque (29). One may not only visualize the cauda equina through the water soluble dye, but partially fibrosed root sheaths are more likely to fill with the less viscous agent. Arachnoiditis is less likely to occur with metrizamide, and persistent postmyelography symptoms are reduced (2). Contrast study of the lumbosacral theca will point to focal disease in the spinal canal or may indicate diffuse adhesive lesions with various degrees of CSF blockage.

Electromyography and Nerve Conduction Velocity

In the hands of an experienced electromyographer, electromyography is often valuable in defining the extent and distribution of nerve and root involvement in a chronic syndrome and particularly in suggesting pure myofascial syndromes that are not secondary to neural mechanisms. These studies are extremely complex in the chronic state; often acute root changes will disappear despite persistent pain, or more diffuse involvement may herald a progressive adhesive process. Specific distal muscles should be sampled for each root suspected and the paraspinal muscle mass tested at each spinal level. Abnormalities in the latter may be the only finding in more subtle cases. Nerve conduction velocities indicate peripheral nerve entrapment or neuropathy. The H-reflex is a convenient tool for identifying pure sensory lesions in the sciatic distribution (39). The reader is referred to specific texts for further information (11). Evolution or resolution of electrical changes during the course of therapy is of primary importance in dealing with neurogenic pain. It is noteworthy that symptoms of neurogenic "ischemia" are intermittent; thus, the electrical studies done to confirm root compromise may be normal in the resting state.

Differential Nerve Block Studies

This technique is based on the work of Gasser and Erlanger, who demonstrated that stimulating a mixed peripheral nerve produces a compound action potential that changes with the varying distances of the stimulating electrode (20). At a suitable distance, A-alpha, A-beta, and A-delta fibers can be separated. Based on that data, peripheral nerve fibers were classified into A, B, and c fibers. Different local anesthetic concentrations have selective sensitivities for A-alpha, A-delta and c fibers (42). This then is the basis for differential spinal and epidural blocks (21,40).

Differential spinal block (traditional technique—antegrade evaluation).

The patient is shown four identical syringes, each containing 10 ml of solution. Syringe 1 contains normal saline, and syringes 2, 3, and 4 contain 0.25% procaine, 0.5% procaine, and 1% procaine, respectively. After a lumbar puncture with a 22-gauge needle, the solution from each syringe is injected at 20-min intervals in the subarachnoid space in the above order. After each injection, the patient is evaluated for subjective relief of pain and objective evidence of (a) sympathetic block (skin temperature, skin resistance, or psychogalvanic reflex changes), (b) sensory block, and (c) motor block. The data obtained is interpreted in the following manner: Objective changes are noted at the time the patient obtains subjective relief of pain. If the patient experiences pain relief after the saline injection and no objective changes are noted, the pain is labeled psychogenic. Relief with 0.25% procaine, with an increase in skin temperature in the lower extremities but without sensory and motor changes, indicates that the pain is transmitted via the c fibers. Pain relief with 0.5% procaine suggests pain transmission via A-delta and c fibers. Relief with 1% procaine blocks larger A fibers and indicates that the pain is caused mostly by muscle spasm or joint pathology. If none of the solutions relieve the patient's pain, the pain is considered to be centrally mediated. This procedure takes about 3 hr to perform and is very uncomfortable for the patient.

Modified differential spinal block (retrograde evaluation).

Recently, a modified differential spinal block was described by Akkineni and Ramamurthy (1). The placebo (saline, 10 ml) is injected first. If the patient's pain is relieved the pain is labeled as psychogenic. If his pain is not relieved, 2 ml of 5% procaine (hyperbaric) is injected. If there is pain relief, the diagnosis is made by evaluating the recovery process. If pain returns with recovery of motor power, then it is transmitted through the A-alpha, A-beta and A-gamma fibers. If it returns with recovery of sensation, then the pain pathway is in A-delta and c fibers, and if pain does not return with recovery of sensation, then the pain pathway is in the c fibers alone.

Differential epidural blocking.

Some authors prefer differential blocking with an epidural technique to prevent postspinal headache and also to have the option of inserting a catheter (48). This allows the patient to be in a comfortable position for evaluation. Both antegrade and retrograde evaluations have been done. One of the authors (P. P. Raj) has evaluated over 500 patients with differential epidural blocks in the past 10 years. For the past 2 years, retrograde differential blocking has been done exclusively (49). In this method, 20 ml of a 3% solution of 2-chloroprocaine is injected via an epidural needle or after an epidural catheter is placed. This volume is needed to ensure that all the lumbosacral nerve roots in the epidural space will be bathed. In patients suspected of having epidural fibrosis or other occlusive pathology, spreading of the local anesthetic in the epidural space is a problem. But this is corrected by inserting a catheter and adding enough of the drug in 5 ml increments until the lumbosacral plexus distribution is adequately blocked. One can then evaluate the pain pathways as the patient is recovering from the block. The table shows the technique of performing a retrograde differential epidural block.

This drug, 2-chloroprocaine, is chosen because of its rapid onset of action and rapid disappearance. Rapid onset permits quick determination of the height and intensity of the block; psychogenic pain can be differentiated from sympathetic or somatic pain at this stage. Rapid disappearance permits assessment of c fiber, A-delta and A-alpha fiber function within 1 hr. Usually only one dose (20 ml) of 2-chloroprocaine is required for retrograde assessment. Rapid elimination of 2-chloroprocaine by plasma cholinesterase facilitates the patient's return to normal physiologic status. This is necessary if the procedure is to be done on an outpatient basis.

Psychologic Evaluation

The Minnesota Multiphasic Personality Inventory (MMPI) is one of the most valid and reliable of personality profile measures for differentiating between patients

TABLE 1. *Retrograde differential epidural block*

| | | | | | Objective findings | | | | | |
| | | | | | Motor power | | | Sensation | Temp °F | |
Time	Medication	BP	Pulse	Subjective feelings	Leg	Knee bend	Toes	Pinprick	R. leg	L. leg
Control		116/65	72	Pain and discomfort in back, L. hip, and L. thigh	✓	✓	✓	✓	86	88
0 min	2-chloroprocaine, 3% 20 ml in epidural space	120/70	76		✓	✓	✓	✓	86	88
10 min		112/70	72	Feelling of warmth, some pain	→	→	✓	→ to T$_9$	89	93
20 min		120/60	72	No pain	→	→	→	→ to T$_6$	92	94
60 min		120/60	72	No pain	✓	✓	✓	→ to T$_9$	96	96
70 min		120/60	72	Some return of pain	✓	✓	✓	✓	90	92
80 min		120/60	72	Return of pain to preblock level	✓	✓	✓	✓	88	89

The results of a differential epidural block in a 45-year-old man with pain in the low back, left hip, and left thigh and a history of four surgical procedures in the lumbar area. Findings showed that the pain was transmitted via A-delta and c fibers. Following the investigative differential blocking, the relief obtained by a series of sympathetic blocks was not enough. Stimulation by percutaneously inserted epidural electrodes gave the patient 70% pain relief. It is important to note that blood pressure and pulse were stable during the differential study. Hypotension may make the test unreliable.

with psychiatric conditions and normal individuals (57). For nonpsychiatric patients, the first three MMPI scales have traditionally been considered the most useful. These comprise the "neurotic triad"—hypochrondriasis, depression, and hysteria. Sternbach (56) described four types of MMPI profiles most frequently encountered in patients with chronic pain. He cautions, however, that the profiles do not permit differentiating psychogenic from somatogenic patients.

1. *Hypochrondriasis Profile*. The patients display extreme somatic preoccupation and are difficult to manage with traditional pain therapies (45).
2. *Reactive Depression Profile*. These are patients with high depression scores who are willing to admit that pain has gotten them down and who respond well to antidepressant medications.
3. *Somatization Profile*. The scores from these patients display a classical "V," with high scores for hypochondriasis and hysteria and low scores for depression. They deny emotional disturbances. They seem to adjust to their pain and derive satisfaction from people feeling sorry for them.
4. *Manipulative Reaction Profile*. The patients have clear physical findings, with an elevated psychopathic deviate scale. They have learned the value of pain behaviors and manipulate others.

More recently, Bradley and associates (6) used a multivariate clustering technique to identify homogenous subgroups among the MMPI scale profiles.

1. *Type A*. These patients have elevations on the first three MMPI scales only. Pain experienced by these patients usually responds to therapy.
2. *Type B*. These patients usually do not have significant elevation on any scale. These patients experience dependency conflicts but remain too highly defended to express them via social or psychologic channels.
3. *Type C*. These patients' MMPIs have elevated scores on the hypochondriasis, depression, hysteria, and schizophrenia scales. These patients are severely neurotic and threatened by emotional interaction.
4. *Type D*. These patients' scores show a conversion "V" similar to that seen in Sternbach's somatization reaction group. This group usually has moderate success in an operant treatment program.

Other psychometric tests used today in patients with chronic pain include the Hathaway and McKinley Test for Degree of Psychopathology, the Cornell Medical Index for Degree of Somatization, the Pilowsky and Spence Questionnaire for Illness Behavior, the State-Trait Anxiety Inventory for Dimensions of Affect; The Zung Scale for Depression, and The Social Readjustment Rating Scale of Rahe for Effect of Environmental Stress (7,24,27,44,54,63).

DIAGNOSIS OF PAIN

After completion of the history, physical examination, and other investigative procedures, a low back pain syndrome can be essentially categorized into one of four groups: neurologic, myofascial, skeletal, or psychogenic. A group of patients, however, will present with combinations of neurologic and myofascial pains, neurologic and skeletal pains, or myofascial and skeletal pains. All these groups usually have an overlay of psychogenic pain behavior (Fig. 6). How can one evolve a management plan that will cater to all these complex syndromes? Perhaps the answer is in looking at the physiologic and psychologic changes that occur as the result of the anatomic pathologies. A mode of therapy is planned that will revert those physiologic and psychologic changes towards normal.

The patient should be cautioned early in the initial examination that total reversion to a normal state cannot reasonably be achieved even by successful therapy; most anatomic changes of chronic pain are fixed, e.g., muscle fibrosis does not disappear even though pain from this structure may be removed. A 50% improvement in pain relief, drug intake, and function is probably a reasonable goal for therapy in chronic pain. This understanding between patient and physician provides a basis for a mutually beneficial relationship. The lack of such realization is behind many failures.

Pathophysiology of Neurogenic Pain

Any "pain" reaching consciousness must by definition involve the nervous system, at least in transmission from the structure of origin, patterns of radiation or referral and ultimately transit through the spinal cord and thalamus to the primary

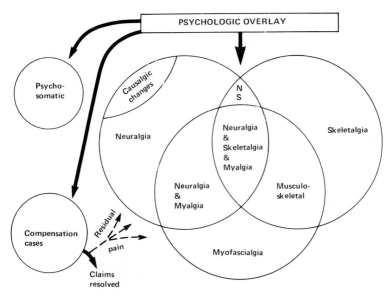

FIG. 6. Schematic showing etiology of pain in chronic low back syndrome. The "pure category" is rare and is seen as the acute manifestation of chronic pain. As the pain becomes chronic, complex syndromes evolve and require varied therapeutic management. NS = Neuroskeletal pain, e.g., facet syndrome, spondylolisthesis.

pain cortex and limbic (interpretive) cortex. However, we limit the term "neural pain" to apply to situations where the nerve root or peripheral nerve itself is compromised and actually inciting the nociceptive stimulus. The involved neural structures are the cauda equina, the spinal roots at the foramina, the dorsal primary rami and facet joint nerves, the lumbosacral plexus in the paravertebral space, and the peripheral nerves. The cauda equina and specific roots at the foramina may be involved intra- or extradurally.

An originally pure neural syndrome often evolves to encompass myofascial complications and a causalgic component, as well as the increasingly complex psychologic modifiers of a chronic pain state. As in the case report above, persistent nerve root pain from arachnoiditis initiates muscle changes from prolonged spasm, which then involves adjacent structures in the gluteal region and the iliotibial tract. The secondary pain structures may remain even after the original root lesion is relieved. Chronic muscle pain then enters the spinal cord through entirely different nerve roots from those originally involved. Reflex sympathetic mechanisms are incited, and the patient experiences a constant burning discomfort, as well as the pain of neural radiation pattern and the myofascial component.

Neural pain that involves the low back is generally referred both below the knee and higher up the axis; all the roots that may be compromised have dermatomal distributions extending below the knee. This is a helpful differential finding in separation of myogenic and skeletogenic categories of pain that are usually more localized to the lumbosacral area or hip or thigh. Nerve root pain, whether in the cauda equina or at the exit foramen, may come from compression or entrapment of the structure, from intermittent ischemia (neurogenic claudication), or from fixed ischemic or neuropathic changes (diabetic, viral, etc.). The neuropathic root hurts at rest, whereas pain from other causes of root irritation may generally be relieved in certain positions.

Facet Syndromes

In this mechanism of pain, chronic irritation of the facet joint is referred as pain by the sinuvertebral nerve twig into the dorsal primary ramus and, hence, into the appropriate sciatic distribution. Patients may have a predominance of back pain or may have sciatica without actual nerve root compression (25,38). The EMG is normal, and mechanical stretching of the sciatic nerve is nondiagnostic. The myelogram does not show root compromise. Diagnostic blocks of the distal dorsal ramus as it passes the facet may be helpful. Radiographs may show hypertrophic facets or may be normal.

Causalgia and Reflex Sympathetic Dystrophy

This probably represents a spectrum of severity involving the same symptoms and perhaps mechanism. True causalgia usually follows partial injury to a major nerve trunk such as the sciatic nerve or its large branches. Reflex dystrophy or minor causalgia is much more common and may occur following the minor trauma to neural structures that accompanies fractures or soft tissue injuries; it is also not unusual as an iatrogenic complication of surgical or neurolytic therapy. Clinical characteristics include burning, poorly localized pain often with a stabbing component, hyperesthesia, and vasomotor and sudomotor alterations leading to ultimate trophic changes that themselves may provide noxious afferent stimuli to compound the syndrome. In causalgia, the pain is generally distal in an extremity with a more proximal injury. An evaluation of possible mechanisms of causalgic pain is given by Bonica (3); he believes that throughout the nervous system, changes of a dynamic nature occur, involving denervation hypersensitivity, initially in the injured peripheral nerve but ultimately involving synaptic activity at all levels.

Lumbosacral plexus involvement in the etiology of pain may be from traction or avulsion injury but more commonly is compressive and caused by tumor or retroperitoneal scarring. This is a difficult area to evaluate. The EMG may be helpful in defining overlapping innervations, and an intravenous pyelogram may show displacement of the ipsilateral ureter indicating anatomic reorganization of the area. Traction injury of the lumbosacral plexus and roots is rare because of the massive musculature that protects the lower extremity from forceful abduction (41).

Peripheral neuropathy must be ruled out in any pain that involves the distal leg, particularly if it does not follow a root distribution. The sensory alteration tends to be nondermatomal (stocking type) and of a causalgic burning nature. Causes are legion and may coexist with any low back syndrome, particularly in an older or malnourished patient who is chronically ill. The nerve conduction velocity is a key diagnostic study; conditions with reduced nerve conduction velocity must be differentiated from peripheral entrapment syndromes.

Pathophysiology of Myofascial Pain

The lower portion of the back with its large muscles and extensive fasciae and ligaments is vulnerable to myofascial pain. Faulty posture is a major cause of low back pain (5). The evolution from the quadruped to upright posture of man has placed great stresses and strains on the lumbosacral myofascial tissues and dorsal muscles. If to these are added further stresses and strains caused by faulty posture, chronic intolerable pain may result.

At first, the postural disturbances are functional and the body tries to compensate for them. If the imbalance persists, the burden shifts to the bones, joints, and ligaments. The anteroposterior curves of the spine become exaggerated, resulting in increased cervical and lumbar lordosis. The force that pulls the lumbar spine foward off the sacrum is increased. Initially, this force is resisted by the facets, the surrounding ligaments, and the overlying muscles. But when this is not enough, the increased stress and strain causes pain and muscle spasm. The muscle spasm produces scoliosis. The weight bearing is transferred from the center of metatarsal arch to the heels, and the feet evert. At this time, the patient assumes the characteristic posture of head protrusion, rounded and drooped shoulders, flat chest, protuberant abdomen and inclined pelvis.

The myofascial pain may be due to one or more of the following causes: (a) reflex muscle spasm, (b) ischemia of the myofascial structures, (c) decreased nutrition, (d) fatigue of the muscle due to excessive use, and (e) muscle injury. In most instances, the mechanism of pain involves an interference with oxidative processes in the muscle caused by a decrease in the supply of oxygen, enzymes, and other nutrients necessary for muscle metabolism.

When fatigue follows overexertion, pain and soreness are experienced hours or days later. These may result from increases in cellular metabolites and water that stimulate nociceptive nerve endings. Once the painful state is produced, it can be perpetuated by feedback cycles from myofascial trigger points (4). Muscle spasm is associated with pain and tenderness of the affected muscles. The pain is constant and diffuse. When a group of muscles is activated by motion, sharp stabbing pain may be experienced. Trigger points that are extremely sensitive to touch and pressure are anatomically located in the muscles. Analgesics and systemic relaxants have no effect on these muscle spasms and the patient becomes restless, irritable, tense, and fatigued. This in turn aggravates the muscle spasm and a vicious cycle ensues.

Low back pain of myofascial origin can be caused by various conditions. These include postural disturbances, degenerative lesions, and myofascial disorders. The myofascial syndromes are the common causes of intolerable pain seen in the pain clinics. They may progress through three stages.

Stage I—Myofascial Syndrome

In patients with stage I myofascial syndrome, only the paravertebral muscles (multifidus and sacrospinalis) are involved. There is tenderness over the lumbar paravertebral region with two trigger points, one midway between T_{12} and the posterior superior iliac spine and the second at the posterior superior iliac spine. Pain is usually bilateral, but there may be more tenderness and spasm on the affected side (Fig. 5). The syndrome is usually seen following acute lumbar injuries in which the patient has recovered but has failed to exercise his back, or after multiple lumbar surgeries.

Stage II—Myofascial Syndrome

Patients with a stage II condition experience tenderness and spasm of the gluteal muscles of the affected side of the lumbar paravertebral muscles in addition to chronic muscle spasm. The tenderness is usually seen in the gluteus medius and minimus and over the greater trochanter. There is no involvement of the sciatic nerve and straight leg raising (SLR) is negative for sciatica. In rare instances, the pyriformis muscle may also be tender, and patients may, in addition, have sciatica resulting from sciatic nerve irritation in the gluteal region. Patients with this myofascial syndrome have difficulty sitting and constantly move around, and they may be bedridden in a fixed lateral posture. This syndrome is seen in patients with primary sacroiliac injury (ligamentous, joint or muscle) or after a bone graft from the iliac crest in patients who have undergone multiple back operations.

Stage III—Myofascial Syndrome

In patients with stage III disease, the chronic muscle spasm and tenderness has progressed from the lumbar paravertebral region to the gluteal muscles and then to the iliotibial tract in the lateral aspect of the thigh. Trigger points can be elicited in the appropriate muscles, including over the posterior superior iliac spine and over the greater trochanter. These patients are usually bedridden and unable to exercise at all.

Pathophysiology of Skeletal Pain

Pain may arise from pathology of the bone, periosteum, ligaments or joints. There are many systemic diseases, e.g., rheumatoid arthritis, that involve these structures, and that have specific treatments. Metastatic tumors frequently involve bone at multiple sites and cause pain by periosteal pressure. There may be pathologic fractures of the spine or diffuse involvement of the pelvic bones, hips, femurs, etc. Often, spinal metastases grow from one vertebral body into the spinal canal and cause neurogenic pain and loss of function. Bone scans with specific radioisotopes are essential additional studies to diagnose these conditions.

Benign skeletal pain as part of the low back syndrome may result from diffuse or focal spondylitic changes in the spine with multiple osteophytes impinging at the foramina or forming bony "bars" that narrow the spinal canal. Facet joint bony changes are frequent. Pseudoarthroses may form after spinal fractures and nonunion or in-fusion masses from previous surgery. Congenital spinal anomalies, such as spondylolysis and spondylolisthesis, cause abnormal ligamentous tension and pain before any nerve root compromise occurs.

The largest group of patients with low back pain are those categorized by spondylogenic skeletal pain. EMGs are negative, and there is usually tenderness to pressure over the facets and increase of pain with spinal manipulation. Segmental instability of the spine may perpetuate pain. Such instability is indicated by the movement of one vertebra on another during a flexion-extension maneuver under radiographic control, and the loss of lordotic posture at the unstable segment. Disk degeneration seldom produces instability.

THERAPEUTIC MANAGEMENT

The therapeutic procedures required in managing patients with low back pain depend on the severity and acuteness of the condition. Acute disabling low back pain, regardless of etiology, requires immediate relief. Once the pain is reduced to a tolerable level, the cause can be ascertained. However, the main principle in managing these patients is to formulate a therapy program that allows each patient to lead a productive life within the limits of his pain.

Therapeutic Options for Acute Intolerable Pain

For acute intolerable pain, the origin must first be determined. If the pain originates in the neural or skeletal tissues, surgical techniques may be indicated. However, nonsurgical modes of therapy should be considered in preference to surgery because of serious postsurgical sequelae in patients with low back pain. The available nonsurgical procedures can be classified as (a) nerve blocks, (b) drug therapy, (c) modulation therapy, (d) physical therapy, and (e) psychotherapy. Nerve blocks are most successful in treating intolerable pain, whereas other modalities could be used for maintenance of relief. If the pain originates in myofascial tissues, then surgery should never be considered. Certainly, subarachnoid and epidural blocks will relieve pain in all tissues distal to the block, but direct myoneural blocking of the involved myofascial tissues is preferred. The trigger points are helpful in this respect. One needs only to block the trigger points with 2 to 3 ml of local anesthetics with or without a steroid. At the University of Cincinnati Pain Control Center, a mixture of 0.75% bupivacaine (for prolonged blocking of afferent pain fibers), 1% etidocaine (for prolonged blocking of efferent fibers), and decadron (4 mg/10 ml) is used with good results. Travell (59) has pointed out, however, that various local anesthetics, as well as dry needling and saline, have been helpful in decreasing the pain of myofascial origin.

Therapeutic Options for Chronic Tolerable Pain

After the acute intolerable pain has been reduced to a tolerable level, one has to consider the options for *continued* pain relief. This has been the hardest task for a pain specialist.

Neurogenic Pain

For neurogenic pain, there are essentially seven options. These include (a) further surgery to decompress roots or nerve, and/or to relieve pain, (sympathectomy, rhizotomy, etc.); (b) injection of steroids (epidural, subarachnoid, nerve root); (c) neurolytic therapy (epidural, subarachnoid, nerve root); (d) electrical blockade (epidural stimulation); (e) administration of drugs; (f) radiofrequency and cryo blocks; and (g) operant conditioning (biofeedback, imagery and relaxation therapy, hypnosis, etc.). They will be discussed in more detail below.

Surgical therapy.

Surgery is initially considered to free the root or nerve from compression or irritation. Probably about 15% of patients who have had surgery for disk disease do not get better and undergo further surgery (10). In the orthopedic literature, much is made of the concept of segmental instability in regard to the indications for fusion of one or more vertebral levels. The fusion may be done after the initial disk excision or at the time of reoperation.

Indications for surgical therapy are based on continued mechanical compromise of roots at the foramina or in the cauda equina, the likelihood that this can be relieved and the correlation of the "anatomic" lesion on contrast studies and EMG with the patient's syndrome (see case report above).

If there is a persistent extradural defect at one or two roots, which are clinically involved, re-exploration may be indicated. In the narrow canal syndrome, wide decompression must be achieved, including a half level above and below the significant myelographic constriction of the thecal sac. Chemical root blocks may give an indication of which roots are mediating pain and aid in planning further decompression surgery. Re-exploration merely to see if something significant can be found is almost always useless and probably detrimental. Even with successful surgical re-exploration, the patient may eventually have return of pain (see case report). After two attempts at surgical cure, other modalities should be tried. The surgical therapy of arachnoiditis is usually of little lasting benefit unless the adhesive process is localized to one root (9,30,47). Generally, it is much more diffuse, often bilateral and additional damage may be done to the delicate rootlets in attempting dissection or lysis of fibrous adhesions. Although there are a few reports that discuss microsurgical lysis of adhesions, overall results are not good enough to warrant the procedure except in an occasional patient.

Surgical procedures to cut nerve fibers have a specific but limited place in pain therapy and should be used only for intractable intolerable pain that has failed to respond to other therapies. The wide range of possible neurologic procedures to control pain are reviewed in detail by Lipton and McLennan (37). Generally, cordotomy is not done for pain of nonmalignant origin because of the liability of postcordotomy dysesthesia that may develop months to years later. Rhizotomies of sensory roots at L_4 through S_1 may be useful if diagnostic blocks show that they will be effective. Again, the return of pain at a later date is not unusual, and the loss of proprioception in the lower extremity is a problem in ambulation. Sacral rhizotomy may be useful in occasional patients who have impaired bladder and bowel function.

Lumbar surgical sympathectomy may be indicated in causalgic pain of the lower portion of the body, particularly in syndromes of recent onset that have responded favorably but transiently to repeated sympathetic blockade (5).

Steroids.

These were used first by Lievre, who injected hydrocortisone into the epidural space (36). Since then, caudal, lumbar epidural, spinal and nerve root injections of a local anesthetic and steroid mixtures have become popular for the conservative management of neurogenic pain.

It is thought that cortocoid preparations act locally, resolving edema and reducing pressure on irritated tissues (14,22,58). It is possible that the beneficial results of epidural steroids may also be due to a systemic effect (32,52). A note of caution here. One should know the other contents of the steroid mixture and limit the injections to a maximum of three. Injections should not be repeated earlier than 2 weeks for fear of steroid "overdose" (Cushing's syndrome) or local neurolytic effect due to picolinium and polyethyleneglycol. The technique at the University of Cincinnati Pain Control Center is as follows: Epidural puncture is made as close as possible to the segmental level of the pain (caudal for sciatica, lumbar for lumbar root involvement). From 10 to 15 ml of a mixture containing 0.25% bupivacaine and 80 mg of methylprednisolone is injected through the needle. A catheter is then placed 1 cm distal to the needle and the needle removed. The patient is turned supine. After 30 minutes, if the pain relief is not adequate, another 10 to 15 ml of the 0.25% bupivacaine and 40 mg of methylprednisolone is injected via the catheter. Back exercises are taught once pain relief is obtained. The procedure can be done on an outpatient basis if adequate facilities are available for monitoring and resuscitation. Results reported by Bromage (8) indicate good relief in 35 to 38% of patients and fair relief in 26 to 31% of patients. Our unpublished data show similar results.

Neurolytic therapy.

Not usually indicated for benign neurogenic pain.

Electrical Blockade and *Drug therapy.*

These topics will be discussed below in the section on musculoskeletal pain.

Radiofrequency and cryoblocks.

Thermal moderation of nerve roots with radiofrequency or cryotherapy is useful in achieving a selective sensory lesion in a mixed nerve. Such procedures may be repeated if necessary. Stimulators accompany the thermal probe and aid in localizing the electrode tip position. Perhaps the most useful therapy for neurogenic pain that cannot be anatomically modified and is too diffuse for specific root therapy is chronic blockade with electrical stimulation proximal to the level of pain origin. This may be achieved transiently by acupuncture and by T.E.N.S. or by implanted epidural electrodes (50).

Musculoskeletal Pain

The relaxed muscle has to be prevented from going back into spasm after the pharmacologic effect of the injected drugs has worn off. The spasm may be precipitated by stretching or contraction of that muscle. Repeat trigger point injections every day are possible but not practical. After three to four such injections, the local anesthetic mixture itself becomes an irritating focus and may cause muscle spasm. Application of a transcutaneous nerve stimulator four times/day for 1 to 2 hr at a time for a 2-week trial period has been extremely beneficial to patients with back pain at the University of Cincinnati Pain Control Center. If the patient continues to improve and has tolerable pain with this regimen in the first 2 weeks, an exercise program is started that is graduated to the patient's tolerance. If the pain becomes intolerable at any point, myoneural blocking is immediately done to bring the pain down to a tolerable level. The main objective is to exercise (stretch and contract) the painful agonistic and antagonistic muscle groups so that they do not go into spasm with normal muscle activity. This stops the barrage of painful impulses that originate from the trigger points. Increasing the exercise level increases the activity and O_2 consumption of the muscles. However, when the muscles are relaxed, an increased blood supply is available to the active muscle fibers and, hence, more nutrition. The increased blood flow also washes out accumulated acid metabolites. Thus, by increasing nutrition, one can keep the muscle from going into spasm. Continued relaxation maintains the increased blood supply and muscle bulk. Both are beneficial to prevent further muscle spasm (4).

Drug therapy.

Drugs should not generally be the keystone in a chronic pain treatment program. Drugs can be beneficial when used discriminately to relieve specific conditions that may otherwise compromise the patient's ability to deal with his basic pain problem. Relatively simple, recently acquired, and uncomplicated back pain problems become iatrogenic disasters because patients fail to receive appropriate advice and treatment at a point at which their condition is easily correctable. Chronic drug use produces no lasting pain relief and adds drug abuse to the patient's list of problems. When short-term use of medication is indicated, one should remember that once pain has been reduced or abated, the agents should be tapered off.

Among the concepts to be considered when managing the patient with chronic back pain is that, although analgesics are important in managing pain problems, they are not complete in themselves. There are only a few relatively and clearly established situations, such as pain from terminal cancer, in which narcotic analgesics should be the primary form of treatment. The most common pain relievers for back pain are the nonsteroid, anti-inflammatory drugs.

Acetaminophen is a good substitute for the nonsteroidal, anti-inflammatory drugs when gastrointestinal problems must be kept to a minimum. However, it is not the drug of choice for chronic low back pain in which inflammation is a prominent feature. In cases of musculoskeletal pain, the combination of chlorozoxazone and acetaminophen has been used widely over the past 20 years. Chlorozoxazone, a benzoxazolone derivative, acts centrally to inhibit reflex acts involved in skeletal muscle spasm. Acetaminophen, a nonsalicylate analgesic agent, acts to provide supplementary pain relief.

Chronic back pain is likely to be associated with either anxiety, hysteria, or reactive depression. The depression involved may be a primary disorder or secondary to environmental stresses or medication excesses. All narcotic analgesics and most minor psychosedatives have the side effect of causing general depression, which can potentiate any tendency for neurotic or psychotic depression. In the patient with chronic low back pain withdrawal from these narcotics and minor psychosedatives often causes enough recovery from depression to eliminate a large percentage of pain complaints. In patients with persistent depression, the antidepressants have proved useful. These agents decrease pain by altering the central appreciation of the quality or intensity of pain (12).

Modulating therapy.

Use of transcutaneous nerve stimulators has now become common in pain management. They have been extremely useful in myofascial pain syndromes. Best results are obtained if the T.E.N.S. is used properly. The experience at the University of Cincinnati Pain Control Center shows that for optimum effect, T.E.N.S. should not be used for more than 2 hours continuously and not more than six times a day. Skin care should be optimal and an appropriate T.E.N.S. should be chosen for each patient. Such stimulation is a useful adjunct to other therapies and cuts down pain medications considerably. In obese patients, T.E.N.S. may not be adequate and one may have to resort to acupuncture, which is qualitatively better since it stimulates subcutaneous nerve endings directly. The disadvantage of acupuncture is that it can only be done by a physician in the Clinic, whereas T.E.N.S. can be used by the patient at home.

Psychotherapy

Biofeedback and relaxation therapy may be used in parallel with myoneural blocking, transcutaneous stimulation, and an exercise program. The important thing is that a management plan is available for each individual patient and the patient knows both what he/she has to do and what to expect from the program. Physical therapy and psychotherapy modalities will be discussed in detail elsewhere in this book.

If the organic factor is not a major element, then the goal of therapy is to change those pain behaviors that interfere with the patient's way of life. Biofeedback, hypnosis, cognitive coping strategies and reinterpretation, operant conditioning, and relaxation techniques and imagery have all been used singly or in conjunction with other therapies for patients with chronic back pain (19,26,51,62). Patients with a reactive depression and somatization profile or a Type D profile respond well, whereas patients with other profiles (hypochondriac and manipulative reactor) have poor results with psychotherapy.

SUMMARY

1. Patients with complex low back pain are referred to the pain clinics.

2. Thorough multidisciplinary pain assessment is necessary for such patients.

3. Identifying the tissue that causes pain helps in planning the management of such patients.

4. Musculoskeletal pain is the common cause of intolerable pain in patients with low back pain.

5. Treatment is directed towards reducing the intolerable pain and improving the strength of affected muscles.

6. Parallel psychotherapy and antidepressive drug therapy is beneficial.

7. Only 50% improvement in subjective pain relief, drug usage, and function can be expected.

8. Modulation therapy with epidural stimulation and cryotherapy are recent additions to the pain therapy armamentarium; results with these techniques will be evaluated with interest.

REFERENCES

1. Akkineni, S. R., and Ramamurthy, S. (1977): Simplified differential spinal block. Abstracts of Scientific Papers, American Society of Anesthesiologists Annual Meeting, p. 765–766.
2. Baker, R. A., Hillman, B. J., McLennan, J. E., et al. (1978): Sequelae of metrizamide myelography in 200 examinations. *Am. J. Roentgen.*, 130:499–502.
3. Bonica, J. J. (1979): Causalgia and other reflex sympathetic dystrophies. In: *Advances in Pain Research and Therapy, Vol. 3*, edited by J. J. Bonica, J. C. Liebeskind, and D. G. Albe-Fessard, pp. 141–166. Raven Press, New York.
4. Bonica, J. J. (1953): General considerations of musculoskeletal pain. In: *Management of Pain*, pp. 1099–1134, Lea and Febiger, Philadelphia.
5. Bonica, J. J.: Regional pains of musculoskeletal origin. In: *Management of Pain*, Lea and Febiger, Philadelphia.
6. Bradley, L. A., Prokop, C. K., Margolis, R., and Gentry, W. D. (1978): Multivariant analyses of the MMPI profiles of low back pain patients. *J. Behav. Med.*, 1:253–272.
7. Brodman, K., Erdmann, A. J., and Wolff, H. G. (1949): Cornell Medical Index Questionnaire. Cornell University Medical College, New York.
8. Bromage, P. R. (1948): *Diagnostic and Therapeutic Applications in Epidural Analgesia*. Saunders, Philadelphia.
9. Burton, C. V. (1978): Lumbosacral arachnoiditis. *Spine*, 3:24–30.
10. Cauchoix, J., Girard, B. (1978): Repeat surgery after disc excision. *Spine*, 3:256–259.
11. Cohen, H. L., and Brumlik, J. (1968): *A Manual of Electromyography*. Hoeber Med. Division, Harper and Row Publ., New York.
12. Dalessio, D. J. (1967): Chronic pain syndromes and disordered cortical inhibition: Effects of tricyclic compounds. *Dis. Nerv. Syst.*, 28:325–328.
13. deValera, E., and Raftery, H. (1976): Lower abdominal and pelvic pain in women. In: *Advances in Pain Research and Therapy, Vol. 1*, edited by J. J. Bonica and D. G. Albe-Fessard, pp. 933–937. Raven Press, New York.
14. Dilke, T. F. W., Burry, H. C., and Grahame, R. (1973): Extradural corticosteroid injection in the management of lumbar nerve root compression. *Br. Med. J.*, 2:635.
15. Donovan-Post, M. J., Brown, M. D., and Gargano, F. P. (1977): The technique and interpretation of lumbar myelograms. *Spine*, 2:214–230.
16. Finneson, B. E. (1973): *Low Back Pain*. J. B. Lippincott Company Publ., Philadelphia, 1973.
17. Finneson, B. E. (1976): Modulating effect of secondary gain on the low back pain syndrome. In: *Advances in Pain Research and Therapy, Vol. 1.*, edited by J. J. Bonica and D. G. Albe-Fessard, pp. 949–952. Raven Press, New York.
18. Fordyce, W. E. (1973): An operant conditioning method for managing chronic pain. *Postgrad. Med.*, 53:123–128.
19. Fordyce, W. E., Fowler, R. S., Lehman, J. F., DeLateur, B. J., Sand, P. L., and Trieschman, R. B. (1973): Operant conditioning in the treatment of chronic pain. *Arch. Phys. Med. Rehabil.*, 54:399–408.
20. Gasser, H. S., and Erlanger, J. (1929): Role of fiber size in establishment of nerve block by pressure or cocaine. *Am. J. Physiol.*, 88:581–591.
21. Gentry, W. D., Newman, M. C., Goldner, J. L., and Balyer, C. von (1977): Relation between graduated spinal block technique and MMPI for diagnosis and prognosis of chronic low back pain. *Spine*, 2:210–213.
22. Goebert, H. W., Jallo, S. J., Gardner, W. J., and Wasmuth, C. E. (1961): Painful radiculopathy treated with epidural injections of procaine and hydrocortisone acetate: Results in 113 patients. *Anesth. Analg. (Cleve.)*, 40:130–134.
23. Gunn, C. C., and Milbrandt, W. E. (1978): Early and subtle low back sprain. *Spine*, 3:267–281.
24. Hathaway, S. R., and McKinley, J. C. (1967): *Minnesota Multiphasic Personality Inventory (Revised)*. Psychological Corp., New York.
25. Hickey, R. F. J., and Tregonning, G. D. (1977): Denervation of spinal facet joints for treatment of chronic low back pain. *N. Z. Med. J.*, 85:96–99.
26. Hilgard, E. R., and Hilgard, J. P. (1975): *Hypnosis in the Relief of Pain*. Kaufman, Los Altos, California.
27. Holmes, T. H., and Rahe, R. H. (1967): The social readjustment rating scale. *J. Psychosom. Res.*, 11:213–218.
28. Hunter, M., Philips, C., and Rachman, S. (1979): Memory for pain. *Pain*, 6:35–46.

29. Irstam, L. (1978): Lumbar myelography with amipaque. *Spine*, 3:70–82.
30. Johnston, J. D. H., and Matheny, J. B. (1978): Microscopic lysis of lumbar adhesive arachnoiditis. *Spine*, 3:36–39.
31. Kirkalady-Willis, W. H., Wedge, J. H., Yong-Hing, K., and Reilly, J. (1978): Pathology and pathogenesis of lumbar spondylosis and stenosis. *Spine*, 3:319–328.
32. Koehler, B. E., Urowitz, M. W., and Killinger, D. W. (1974): The systemic effects of intra-articular corticosteroid. *J. Rheumatol.*, 1:117–125.
33. Leavitt, F., Garron, D. C., D'Angelo, C. M., and McNeil, T. W.(1979): Low back pain in patients with and without demonstrable organic disease. *Pain*, 6:191–200.
34. Lee, C. K., Hansen, H. T., and Weiss, A. B. (1978): Developmental lumbar spinal stenosis: Pathology and surgical treatment. *Spine*, 3:246–255.
35. Lewis, C. S. (1945): *The Problem of Pain*. Macmillan, New York.
36. Liévre, J. A., Bloch-Michel, H., Pean, G., and Uro, J. (1953): L'hydrocortisone en injection locale. *Rev. Rhum. Maladies Osteoartic.*, 20:310.
37. Lipton, S., and McLennan, J. (1980): Neural Blockade. In: *Clinical Anesthesia and Management of Pain*, pp. 679–690. J. B. Lippincott Co., Philadelphia.
38. Lora, J., and Long, D. (1976): So-called facet denervation in the management of intractable back pain. *Spine*, 1:121–126.
39. Magladery, J. W., and McDougall, D. B. (1950): Electrophysiological studies of nerve and reflex activity in normal man. *Bull. Johns Hopkins Hosp.*, 86:265.
40. McCollum, D. E., and Stephen, C. R. (1964): Use of graduated spinal anesthesia in the differential diagnosis of pain of the back and lower extremities. *S. Med. J.*, 57:410.
41. McLennan, J. E., McLaughlin, W. T., Skillicorn, S. A. (1973): Traumatic lumbar nerve root meningocele. *J. Neurosurg.*, 39:528–532.
42. Nathan, P. W., and Sears, T. A. (1961): Some factors concerned in differential nerve block by local anesthetics. *J. Physiol. (Lond.)*, 157:565–580.
43. Nathan, P. W. (1977): Pain. *Br. Med. Bull.*, 33:149–156.
44. Pilowsky, I., and Spence, N. D. (1975): Patterns of illness behavior in patients with intractable pain. *J. Psychosom. Res.*, 19:279–287.
45. Pilowsky, I. (1968): The response to treatment in hypochondriacal disorders. *Austr. N. Z. J. Psychiatry*, 2:88–94.
46. Prieto, E. J., Hopson, L., Bradley, L. A., Byrne, M., Geisinger, K. F., Midax, D., and Marchisello, P. J. (1980): The language of low back pain: factor structure of the McGill Pain Questionnaire. *Pain*, 8:11–19.
47. Quiles, M., Marchisello, P. J., and Tsairis, P. (1978): Lumbar adhesive arachnoiditis—etiologic and pathologic aspects. *Spine*, 3:45–50.
48. Raj, P. P. (1977): Sympathetic pain mechanisms and management. Paper presented at the Second Annual Meeting of the American Society of Anesthesiologists, Hollywood, Florida, March 10–11.
49. Raj, P. P. (1979): Case history 2: nesacaine for retrograde differential epidural blocking, Nesacaine (Chloroprocaine Hydrochloride). In: *Case Studies in Obstetrical and Surgical Regional Anesthesia*, pp. 8–12. Pennwalt Corp., New York.
50. Richardson, R. R., Siqueira, E. B., and Cerullo, L. J. (1979): Spinal epidural neurostimulation for treatment of acute and chronic intractable pain: initial and long term results. *Neurosurgery*, 5:344–348.
51. Rybstein-Blinchik, E. (1979): Effects of different cognitive strategies on the chronic pain experience. *J. Behav. Med.*, 2:93–101.
52. Shuster, S., and Williams, I. A. (1961): Adrenal suppression due to intra-articular corticosteroid therapy. *Lancet*, 2:171.
53. Simons, D. G. (1976): Electrogenic nature of palpable bands and "jump sign" associated with myofascial trigger points. In: *Advances in Pain Research and Therapy, Vol. 1*, edited by J. J. Bonica and D. G. Albe-Fessard, pp. 913–918. Raven Press, New York.
54. Spielberger, C. D., Gorsuch, R. L., and Lushene, R. E. (1970): *STAI Manual for the State-Trait Inventory*. Consulting Psychologists Press, Palo Alto, California.
55. Sternbach, R. A. (1973): Psychological aspects of pain and the selection of patients. *Clin. Neurosurg.*, 21:323–333.
56. Sternbach, R. A. (1974): Aspects of chronic low back pain. *Pain Patients: Traits and Treatment*. Academic Press, New York.

57. Sternbach, R. A., Wolf, S. R., Murphy, R. W., and Akeson, W. H. (1973): Psychosomatics 14:52–56.
58. Swerdlow, M., and Sayle-Creer, W. (1970): A study of extradural medication in relief of the lumbosciatic syndrome. *Anaesthesia*, 25:341–345.
59. Travell, J. (1976): Myofascial trigger points: clinical view. In: *Advances in Pain Research and Therapy*, *Vol. 1*, edited by J. J. Bonica and D. G. Albe-Fessard, pp. 919–926. Raven Press, New York.
60. Waring, E. M., Weisz, G. M., Bailey, S. I. (1979): Predictive factors in the treatment of low back pain by surgical intervention. In: *Advances in Pain Research and Therapy*, *Vol. 3*, edited by J. J. Bonica, J. C. Liebeskind, and D. G. Albe-Fessard, pp. 939–942. Raven Press, New York.
61. Weinstein, P. R., Ehni, G., Wilson, C. B. (1977): *Lumbar Spondylosis*. Year Book Medical Publishers, Chicago.
62. Weinstock, S. A. (1973): A tentative procedure for the control of pain: migraine and tension headaches. In: *Biofeedback and Self Control*, edited by D. Shapiro, T. X. Barber, L. V. DiCara, J. Kamiya, N. E. Miler, and J. Stoyva, pp. 510–512. Aldine Publishing Co., Chicago.
63. Zung, W. W. K. (1965): A self-rating depression scale. *Arch. Gen. Psychiatry*, 12:63–70.

Chronic Low Back Pain, edited by
M. Stanton-Hicks and Robert Boas.
Raven Press, New York © 1982.

The Radiologic Evaluation of Back Pain

David J. Berg

*Special Procedures Section, Department of Radiology, Phoenix General Hospital,
Phoenix, Arizona 85015*

The large number of diagnostic modalities attest to the fact that evaluation of low back pain and sciatica is a difficult and complex task. Other authors, in this volume and elsewhere, have clearly pointed out the significance and prevalence of this malady along with the tremendous impact on both the individual and the economy (30). This presentation will provide an overview of the various radiologic diagnostic parameters available, their usefulness, and a suggested step-wise plan for their implementation.

A schematic diagram of the spinal canal (Fig. 1) provides a guide of the important nerves related to the bony structures. This shows the various areas where nerve

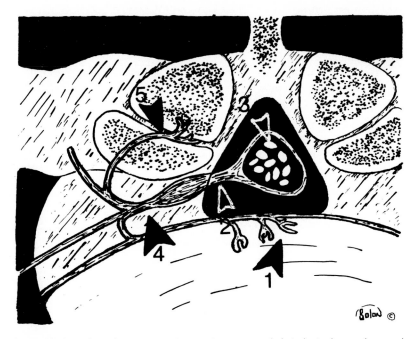

FIG. 1. Various sites where nerve entrapment may occur. **1.** Anterior to dura and nerve sleeves (sinuvertebral and spinal nerves from disk). **2.** Medial part of nerve canal (spinal nerves). **3.** Posterolateral part of main canal (cauda equina from encroaching posterior joints). **4.** Lateral canal recess (spinal and sinuvertebral nerves from prominent superior articular processes). **5.** Facet joints (medial branches of the posterior primary rami).

101

entrapment may occur and explains why diagnosis is difficult. A number of different etiologies may be responsible; these include central bony spinal stenosis, herniated nucleus pulposus, lateral recess compromise, and facet joint abnormalities. These are in addition to the more obvious causes, such as trauma, infection, neoplasms, ankylosing spondylitis, or instabilities from congenital anomalies. Because of the difficulty of imaging this complex anatomical region, it becomes increasingly important that the referring physician carefully assesses the patient and organizes the findings. Obvious referred pain and differentiation of low back pain from radicular pain should be apparent in most cases. This separation will allow the proper imaging modality or at least the proper planned approach to be selected initially.

The available radiologic procedures may be separated into three categories to organize our thinking (Table 1). This grouping has been devised because utilization varies with the expertise of the radiologist and the availability of the equipment. This becomes especially important for the more expensive and regulated angiographic and computerized apparatus. Although availability and experience may ultimately alter the order of use, at the present time most diagnoses of low back pain or sciatica are made by conventional procedures, i.e., plain film radiographs, myelography, radionuclide bone scans, or some combination of all three.

The increasing number of diagnostic tests and their concomitant growing expense coupled with the ever increasing demands of third party and governmental bodies command that a more streamlined systematic approach be used when evaluating back pain. Also, the need to avoid unnecessary surgery is paramount because of the often subsequent disability.

The radiation dose to the patient for each test must also be kept in mind, particularly with younger patients. It has been determined that standard anteroposterior, lateral, and oblique projections of the lumbar spine result in a mean skin dose of 11,319 mR (mC/Kg) (2,28) with a bone marrow dose of 444 mR (666 μ Gy[1]) (36). By comparison, a three-view lumbosacral spine examination produces the same amount of irradiation to the ovaries (238–715 mR) as would a chest radiograph

TABLE 1. *Available radiologic procedures*

Conventional
  Plain films: static and dynamic
  Radionuclide bone scans
  Myelography
Supplemental
  Epidural venography
  Computerized tomography
  Angiography
Controversial
  Diskography
  Epidurography

[1]Gy = Gray.

performed daily for 6 (42), 16 (2), or 98 (3) years (17). Lumbar spine computerized tomography (CT) examination results in 6R (0.06 Gy) per examination (7). Newer generation CT scanners should further decrease the radiation dose per examination as columators and detectors improve.

The sensitivity and specificity of each of the many tests becomes an additional problem. Van Damme (41) compared the diagnostic accuracy of the clinical examination, plain X-ray evaluation, electromyography, myelography, and lumbar phlebography, but unfortunately not of CT scanning. The high false-negative rate of plain X-ray evaluation (31%), clinical examination (14%), and myelography (16%) is distressing. The low false-positive rate of plain X-ray examination (9%) and low false-negative rate for lumbar phlebography (4%) is meaningful and will be discussed below. This study underscores the importance of continued evaluation when the initial X-ray findings are normal, a history of drug abuse is obtained, persistent localized pain is present, or progressive neurologic deficit occurs.

Holmes and Rothman (18) have addressed these problems and have devised a scheme for dealing with lumbar disk disease (Table 2). This algorithm, a set of rules for solving a particular problem in a definite number of steps, separates those patients with cauda equina syndrome or progressive weakness for aggressive early diagnosis and treatment. The remaining patients follow a more conservative course, in which treatment is implemented with step-wise radiographic evaluation used in a logical manner (see ref. 18 for a detailed discussion). Various institutions may need to modify this plan as their particular situation dictates; nevertheless, this represents an excellent and workable plan.

A shortened plan of radiographic evaluation for purposes of this discussion is shown in Table 3. This suggests an approach that considers each modality in relation to the others and employs invasive procedures only when less invasive investigations have been unrewarding.

The primary division follows the Pennsylvania Plan when true motor weakness is present and delay in diagnosis and treatment is unwarranted. In this situation, the recommended course consists of plain films to rule out the obvious causes, followed by myelography or high resolution CT if available, then surgery if indicated. Epidural venography may be substituted for myelography, especially if an L5-S1 disc is suspected because venography is most accurate at this level. Epidurography and/or diskography have a controversial role if all other tests are normal but may be helpful in selected cases.

The plan suggests that in the remainder of patients with low back pain the workup should proceed with plain radiographs followed by radionuclide bone scans. This generally reveals the non-discogenic serious causes, including early ankylosing spondylitis, infection, and neoplasm. Less than 1% of patients with back pain have one of these three as the underlying cause of their pain (12). CT scanning is recommended before myelography to rule out such entities as bony spinal stenosis, undetected lateral recess compromise, facet hypertrophy, occult neoplasms, or postoperative bony hypertrophy. Metrizamide myelography, used last in this clinical

TABLE 2. *Pennsylvania Hospital disk degeneration algorithm*

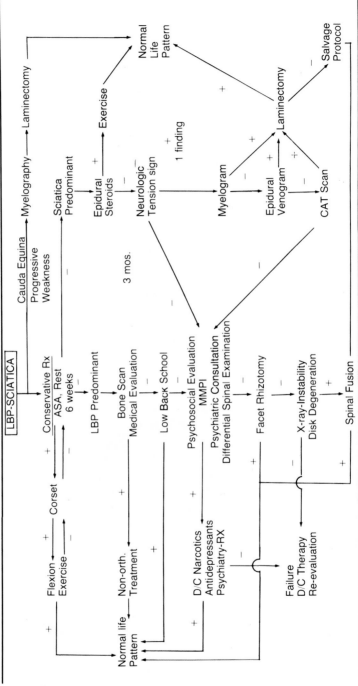

Reprinted from Holmes and Rothman (18) with permission.

TABLE 3. *Schematic for diagnostic work-up of back pain and sciatica*

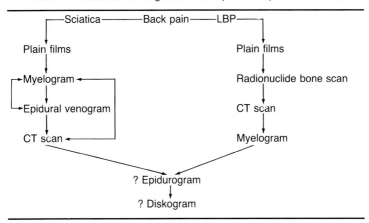

setting, may also be combined with CT as a single examination to aid visualization of the soft tissues within the spinal canal in difficult cases.

Below is a discussion of each modality and several examples of each to ascertain their value and application.

PLAIN RADIOGRAPHIC STUDIES

The standard anteroposterior (AP), lateral, and oblique projections are the most widely used in screening the lumbosacral spine. Spot films coned to the lumbosacral junction, angled AP, and oblique views of the sacroiliac joints may supplement the standard views if clinically indicated. Recently the cost effectiveness of the oblique and coned down L5-S1 lateral projections have been questioned (11,31,33). Table 4 shows the findings that may be obtained from these plain films. These views allow assessment of alignment, vertebral body size comparison, bone density, and architecture, along with gross evaluation of soft tissue structures.

Readily apparent in these studies are cases of ankylosing spondylitis with the bamboo spine appearance (Fig. 2), spondylolisthesis with a marked defect of the pars interarticulares (Fig. 3), and loss of the disk space and sclerosis of the adjoining end-plates resulting from tuberculosis (Fig. 4). Fractures, anomalies, destructive neoplasms, and scoliosis are also generally apparent. Short-leg and pelvic-tilt abnormalities may be demonstrated if weight-bearing films are obtained.

The standard plain films may also be supplemented with complex motion tomography or laminography to improve assessment of intraosseous lesions or anatomical relationships in fracture cases. Unfortunately, there are limitations and disadvantages with laminography because of the significant radiation exposure and the need to move the patient for difficult views. This is frequently hazardous and painful. Difficulty in obtaining adequate detail of the posterior neural arch and the

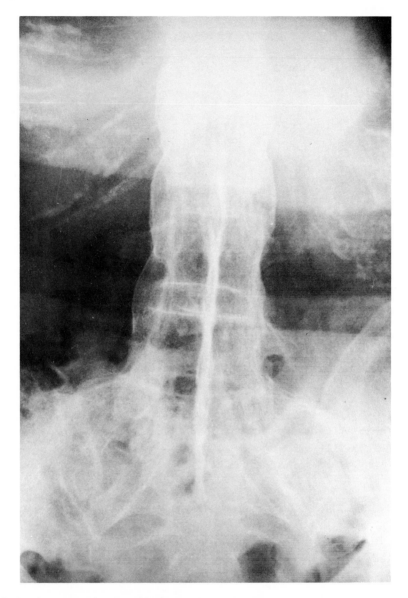

FIG. 2. Anteroposterior view of lumbosacral spine in patient with ankylosing spondylitis. Extensive bony bridging across disk spaces and sacal-iliac joints is apparent.

absence of soft tissue detail adjacent and within the spinal canal are likewise significant drawbacks that are eliminated with CT scanning.

The finding of traction spurs along with disk-space narrowing, loss of lordosis, or abnormal movement may be highly suggestive of disk disease, but all findings should be carefully evaluated. Studies have shown poor correlation between back pain

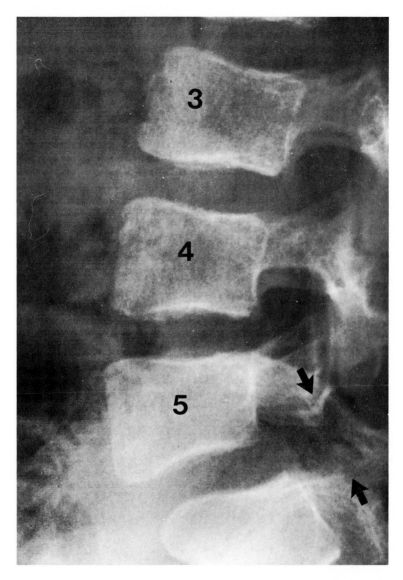

FIG. 3. Lateral view of lumbosacral spine showing anterior subluxation of L5 on S1 with prominent pars interarticulares defect (→) of spondylolisthesis.

and many of the radiologic findings, such as old compression fractures, Schmorl's node, degenerative osteophytes, spina bifida occulta, and spondylosis (13,14,26,27,37,38).

RADIONUCLIDE SCANS

Bone-seeking compounds tagged with radioactive agents are injected intravenously for this procedure. Detectors show the areas of uptake of radioactivity, which

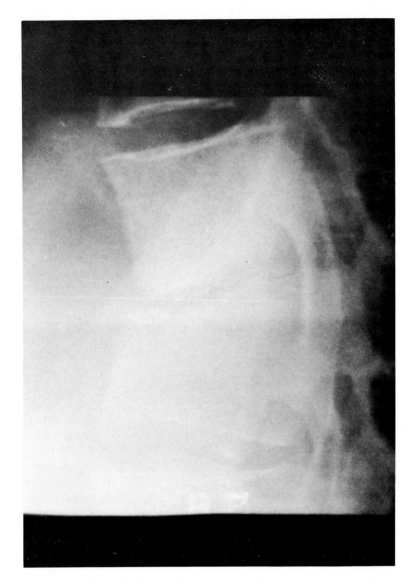

FIG. 4. Coned down lateral view showing narrowed to absent disk space and collapse and sclerosis of adjacent end-plates with resultant kyphotic deformity, resulting from chronic tuberculosis.

are a reflection of bone activity and new bone growth. Technetium is the most commonly used agent at present. In Fig. 5, a scan of a patient with back pain, numerous focal black areas on the skeleton represent the concentration of radioactivity in the multiple prostatic osteoblastic metastatic lesions. Radiographs of the focal abnormalities will confirm the nuclear scan findings and are necessary to

TABLE 4. *Radiographic signs*

Disk-space narrowing
Vacuum disk–Knuttson phenomena
Traction spur
To-and-fro motion with dynamic studies
Absence or reversal or lordotic curve
Scoliosis, pelvic tilt, short leg, congenital anomalies
Bone destruction, sclerosis, expansion
Fracture and dislocation
Paraspinal mass

differentiate them from fractures or degenerative changes since scanning is quite sensitive but is not specific.

Radionuclide bone scans are far more sensitive in detecting early bone lesions because nearly 50% destruction of cancellus bone is needed before a lytic process is radiographically apparent. This suggests that bone scans should replace radiographs as the primary study in almost all cases of suspected metastatic disease and totally in most cases of suspected primary neoplasm. Radiographs should be used in suspicious areas and may be helpful when treatment has been rendered and bone healing has produced sclerosis or in purely lytic lesions, such as multiple myeloma. Early inflammatory infectious conditions and Paget's disease are also easily detected with bone scans.

MYELOGRAPHY

In 1919, the door to myelography was opened by Walter Dandy's (9,10) introduction of air-contrast into the spinal canal. Attention was firmly focused on the intervertebral disk and nerve root irritation a short time later by Mixter and Barr (29) with their description of nucleus pulposus protrusion. Since the introduction in 1944 of ethyliodophenylumdeoylate (Pantopaque), an iodinated ester, most myelography has been performed with this agent.

Various water soluble agents have been tried over the years, beginning with methiodal sodium (Abrodil, Kontrast U) introduced by Arnell and Lidström in 1931 (4). Meglumine iothalamate (Conray meglumine) and meglumine iocarnate (Dimer-X), introduced in 1963 and 1968, respectively, were improvements but had significant limitations because of their neurotoxicity.

In 1968, a nonionic water soluble contrast medium, metrizamide (Amipaque), was developed. Following extensive clinical trials, it was released in 1978 by the Food and Drug Administration for general use in the United States. Despite its limited neurotoxicity, its judicious use with proper attention to technique has allowed it to all but replace Pantopaque as the agent of choice for lumbar myelography. Pantopaque remains useful in cases of spinal block (Fig. 6) where the upper and lower margins need to be established and the contrast should be left in place for posttherapy follow-up studies so that repeated lumbar punctures are avoided. Unusually large patients or those with contraindications for metrizamide still require

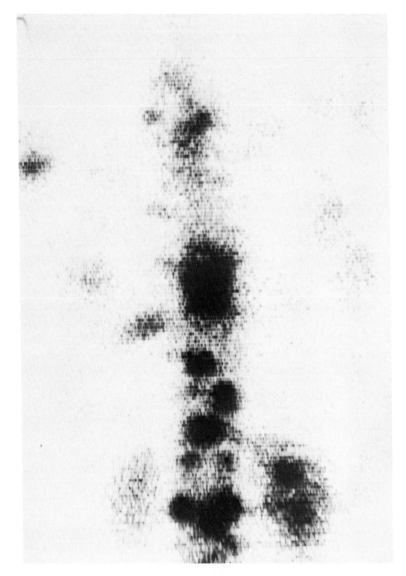

FIG. 5. Radionuclide Tc99m-DP bone scan. Note the multiple areas of increased radioactivity from prostatic metastasis.

Pantopaque. The reader is referred to an excellent work by Sachett and Strother (34) on the specifics and techniques for using metrizamide.

Strict adherence to the manufacturer's recommendations are suggested, especially the need to make sure that patients are well hydrated, are not taking phenothiazines, and are free of liver, renal, or seizure disorders. Chronic alcoholics should not be

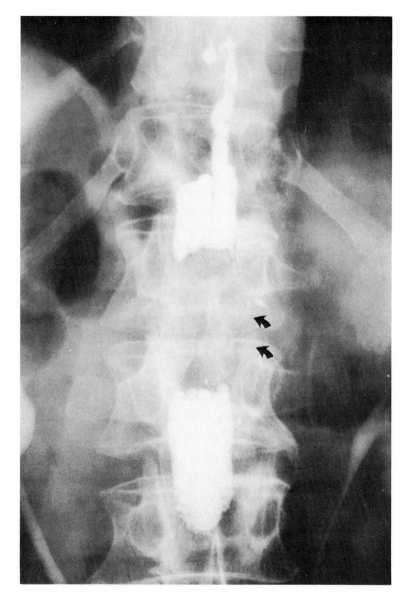

FIG. 6. Pantopaque myelogram showing upper and lower margins of spinal block from lung tumor metastasis. Note loss of left inferior facet of L1. (↖).

given metrizamide, and all attempts should be made to keep large doses out of the head region. Phenobarbitol is the drug of choice for premedication.

Myelography with Pantopaque clearly shows large extradural defects, such as that from a herniated disk at the L5-S1 level (Fig. 7). The more laterally located or subtle lesions compressing only the nerve root sleeve are more easily seen by

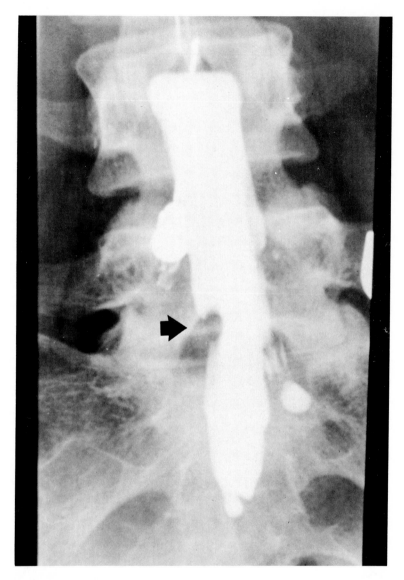

FIG. 7. Pantopaque myelogram showing a large extradural defect (→) at the left L4–5 inter-vertebral level from disk herniation that compresses the entire subarachnoid space.

the less viscous metrizamide as sleeve cut-off. This is shown in Fig. 8, where normal filling is seen above and below and on the contralateral side from the right L4-5 lateral disk protrusion. This finding correlated with the patient's right-sided radiculopathy, and a disk was surgically removed. Asymmetrical axillary pouch filling does not carry the same significance when the oily viscous contrast is used.

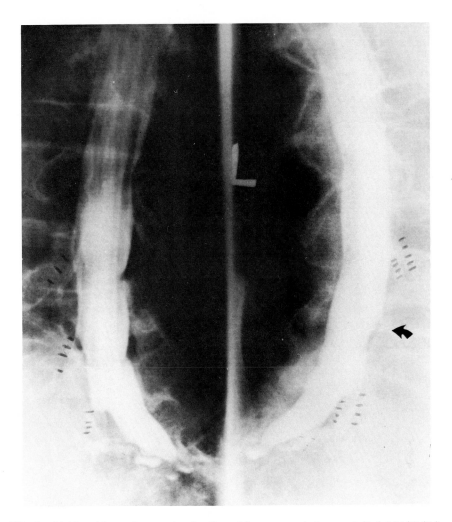

FIG. 8. Metrizamide myelogram showing the subtle nerve root sleeve cutoff of right L5 (↖), which indicates compression from a lateral disk herniation. Note excellent filling of all other nerve root sleeves (markings). The lateral projection was normal.

Figure 9 demonstrates a distinct advantage derived from using the water soluble agent. The myelogram is from a patient who had surgery with subsequent progressive back pain. Metrizamide myelography not only shows the extensive arachnoiditis but also allows use of a small (22-gauge) needle and eliminates the need to remove the agent. In addition, since arachnoiditis has not been associated with the use of metrizamide, no aggravation of this condition by this substance may be expected, in contrast to the use of Pantopaque, where this is a known problem (6). Anyone who has experienced difficulty in removing Pantopaque following mye-

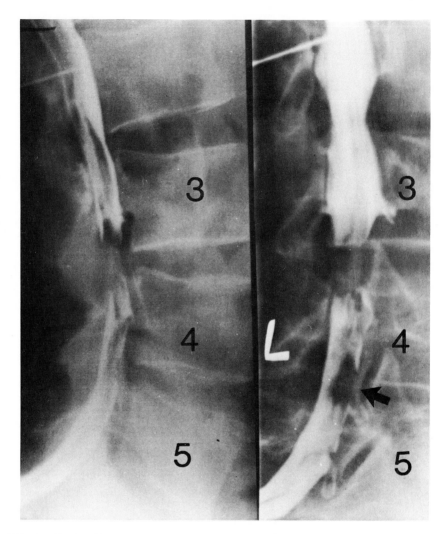

FIG. 9. Metrizamide myelogram showing gross distortion of the entire subarachnoid space with adhesion of the space at L3–4 and simulated focal intradural extramedullary lesion on right L4–5 level (←).

lography can readily appreciate this advantage. On the other hand, metrizamide may also be withdrawn if it is concentrated in a focal area. In addition, supplemental CT studies may follow the metrizamide myelogram immediately or within 3 to 4 hours without loss of information.

When performing myelography, one must always keep in mind, as was pointed out by McRae (27), that disk protrusion may occur in the asymptomatic patient. This finding is not uncommon; those who regularly do cervical myelography frequently note numerous large defects in the asymptomatic lumbar area. Therefore,

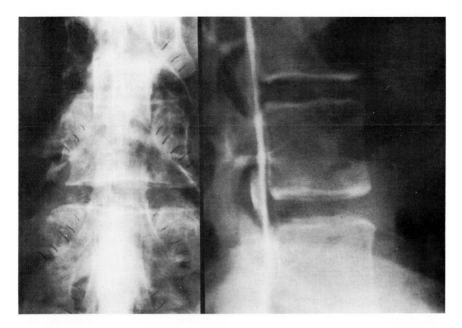

FIG. 10. Epidurogram with both epidural and subarachnoid filling. Note the length of nerve sleeve filling extending past each pedicle. Compare this to the normal subarachnoid filling seen in Fig. 8. Markings were added to outline the sleeve filling.

the clinical findings remain paramount in order to utilize the radiographic findings accurately.

EPIDUROGRAPHY

This technique, puncturing the epidural sac with a needle and introducing air, was first described by Sanford and Doub in 1941 (35). The use of positive contrast was reported in 1963 (25) and again in 1975 (23), with improved visualization of the epidural space and nerve root sleeves for delineating the pressure effect from disk protrusion. A recent report on the use of selective catheterization with contrast injection (32) points out the difficulty that others have encountered with this procedure. Its use is suggested where myelography is equivocal or normal, especially where the L5-S1 epidural space is wide. Although encouraging reports are intermittently found in the literature, this technique has not been widely used over the years.

Figure 10 shows contrast in both the epidural and subarachnoid spaces in this normal study. Excellent filling of the nerve root sleeves is demonstrated.

DISKOGRAPHY

Diskography is performed by percutaneous placement of opaque contrast media directly into the intervertebral disk space via a spinal needle. The pain response

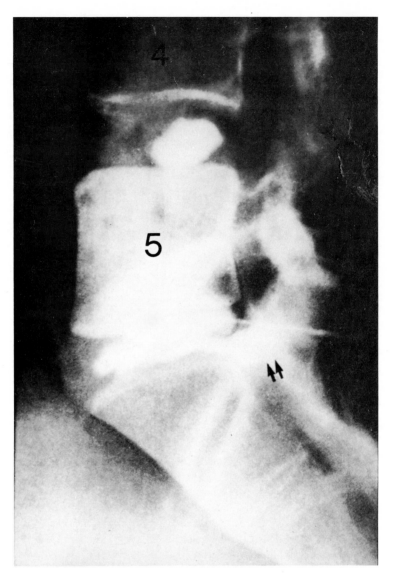

FIG. 11. Diskogram at two levels showing the isolated well-contained, biconcave appearance of the normal L4–5 space. Note elongation of contrast pocket and extravasation into the canal from the degenerated L5–S1 disk (↑ ↑).

during injection, the configuration of the injected materials, and the presence of abnormal contrast extravasation from the contained space are all carefully measured. This was initially described by Lindblom in 1948 (24). The first use of this procedure in the United States was reported in 1951 by Wise and Weiford (44) at the Cleveland Clinic, where it has continued to be a chief diagnostic modality.

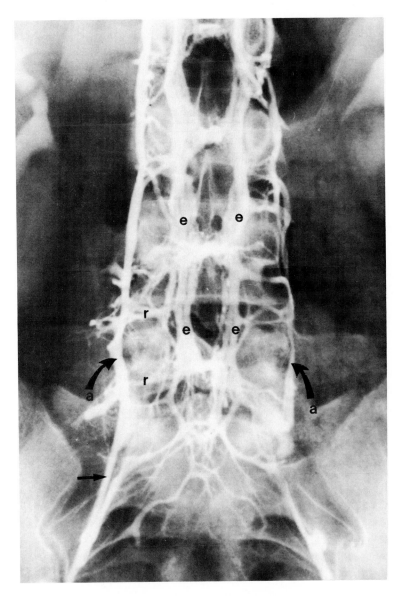

FIG. 12. Normal epidural venous plexus filling. Note catheter in right femoral vein (→); ascending lumbar veins (↗ **a** ↖); anterior epidural veins forming figure 8 patterns (**e**); radicular branches above and below each pedicle (**r**); and symmetrical uniform filling.

Its recommended use is similar to that of epidurography, although it has also been the primary examination for disk disease to the exclusion of myelography. There are, however, significant false positives and negatives, whose incidence is increased if the technique is done with too much sedation or with general anesthesia.

In a much criticized study by Holt (19), 30 prisoners without a history of back pain were examined by this procedure, and many of the diskograms were found to be abnormal. As a result, Holt concluded that the procedure was unreliable. Despite numerous studies and many years of use, diskography remains controversial and, like epidurography, is not a widely used diagnostic tool.

In Figure 11, note the normal biconcave appearance of the L4-5 disk space compared with the elongated appearance of the degenerated L5-S1 disk. Also, note the extravasation of contrast posteriorly into the canal.

EPIDURAL VENOGRAPHY

Epidural venography, initially performed by spinous process intraosseous injection, opacifies the epidural venous plexus (the so-called Batson's plexus). This technique reveals when the veins lying against the posterior longitudinal ligament are compressed by disk protrusion. Fortunately, in 1974, this painful technique was revised by the discovery by Gargano, Meyer and Sheldon (15) that the ascending lumbar and radicular veins could be selectively catheterized via the femoral vein. This catheter technique is relatively simple and safe; it has a reported accuracy equal to and, at the lumbosacral level, superior to Pantopaque myelography. Further studies are necessary, but venography will probably be comparable in accuracy with metrizamide myelography.

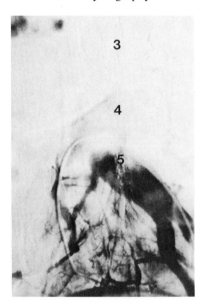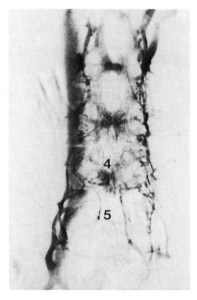

FIG. 13 (left). Epidural venogram showing catheter crossing from left to right and injection into right presacral vein. Note complete cessation of cephalad flow at L4–5 with reflux filling into common femoral vein.

FIG. 14 (right). Venous injection into left L4–5 radicular branch, in same patient as in Fig. 13. Note cessation of caudal flow from injection resulting from a large compressing disk at this level.

Figure 12 is a normal study in a patient with a normal metrizamide myelogram but with an unusually wide lumbosacral epidural space. Excellent filling of the epidural venous plexus shows the central figure 8's of the paired anterior epidural veins, the lateral vertical ascending lumbar veins, and the short horizontal connecting radicular branches above and below each vertebral pedicle.

Figures 13 and 14 are subtraction studies of two separate venous injections. The subtraction is a photographic maneuver done after the study is completed to eliminate the overlying bone and leave only the injected contrast for improved visualization of the smaller veins and any anatomical abnormalities. In this case, complete obstruction to venous filling at the L4-5 level caused by disk herniation and subsequent venous compression is apparent. This shows that in some instances separate injections at different locations are necessary to effect filling above, below, and contralateral to a suspected defect. This technique will prevent many otherwise false-positive studies. Another suggested technique is to perform simultaneous injections through two catheters, one on each side. This, however, necessitates bilateral femoral vein punctures. A distinct advantage of lumbar phlebography is the absence of subarachnoid puncture. This may, in selected cases, also be done on an outpatient basis. Intravenous pressures may be concomitantly measured through the catheter (see Boas, *this volume*).

The low false-negative rate of venography, as shown by the Van Damme study cited above, indicates the high confidence level that may be attained from a normal

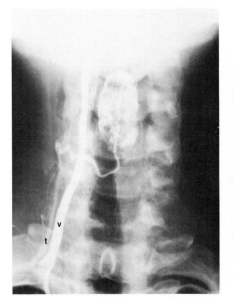 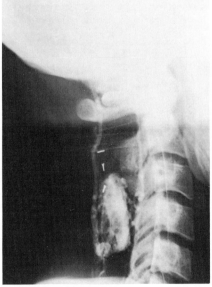

FIG. 15 (left).   AP projection of spine during right subclavian artery contrast injection showing vessels from cervical branches of thyrocervical trunk and vertebral arteries filling the ovoid vascular hemangioblastoma.

FIG. 16 (right).   Lateral projection of hemangioblastoma tumor. Note vascular surgical clips from previous unsuccessful surgery.

study. The reliability of a normal examination allows the following guidelines for use of venography: (a) following normal or equivocal myelography, particularly where a wide lumbosacral epidural space or short caudal sac are present; (b) if strong clinical evidence for a L5-S1 disc is present (venography may be the only examination needed); (c) when the patient refuses myelography or it is contraindicated; (d) when clinical factors necessitate ruling out the presence of a herniated disk; myelography can thus be avoided.

The procedure is contraindicated in patients with known iodine hypersensitivity who cannot be desensitized with steroids—as is any examination that involves halogenated contrast medium. It is also ruled out in patients who have had a previous laminectomy at the suspected level because surgery generally destroys the venous plexus at that location. Other levels or the contralateral side may still be examined. The final limitation of the procedure relates to the skill of the vascular radiologist because interpretation is sometimes difficult.

ANGIOGRAPHY

The introduction of intraarterial contrast by selective catheterization has relatively limited application forback pain. It is primarily used for delineating arteriovenous malformations and indicating the blood supply of vascular tumors and their etiology.

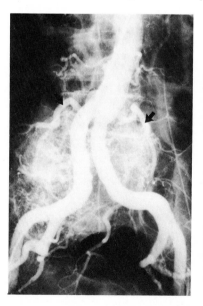 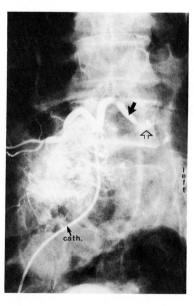

FIG. 17 (left). Aortogram showing prominent lumbar arteries (↓) feeding extensive vascular renal clear cell carcinoma metastasis in the spine.

FIG. 18 (right). Selective catheterization of lumbar artery on right with contrast filling a portion of the renal metastic tumor. Note contrast remaining in left lumbar artery from earlier embolization (↙), coil wires occluding the vessel (⇑), and absence of contrast filling of tumor on the left after the occlusion.

Such a case of recurrent hemangioblastoma in the cervical cord is shown in Figs. 15 and 16; here the major blood supply emanates from the right vertebral artery and branches off the thyrocervical trunk.

Another example of arterial catheter use is transcatheter embolization of arteries that supply painful body metastatic lesions that are resistant to other forms of treatment. Figures 17 and 18 demonstrate the use of this technique for the successful palliation of a pain in a 60-year-old male with metastatic renal clear cell carcinoma who was bedridden and on large doses of narcotics for intractable pain. A large vascular mass representing the tumor is seen initially by abdominal aortography. Here the dilated feeding lumbar arteries are apparent. Figure 18 shows the results after the left lumbar artery was occluded with coil wires.[2] The catheter has been placed into the right side for selective filming of the remaining tumor blush. Residual contrast remains in the left side indicating arterial occlusion.

Generally, angiography is a final definitive study coupled with possible therapy via embolization of tumors and arteriovenous malformations, to be performed by the interventional radiologist. Interventional radiology is now a growing subspecialty.

COMPUTERIZED TOMOGRAPHY

The most recent and undoubtedly one of the most important advances added to the diagnostic armamentarium is computerized tomography (CAT, CT, CT scan-

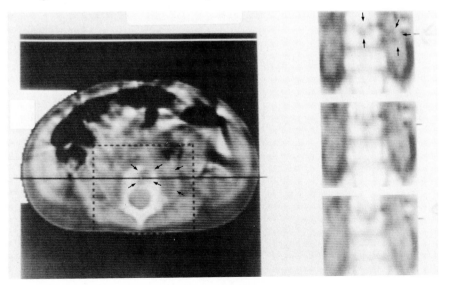

FIG. 19. CT scan of axial view (left) and three coronal reconstructed slices (right). Note the low density defect in the vertebra ( ) and left psoas muscle ( ) from the abscess.

---

[2]Cook Company, Bloomington, Indiana.

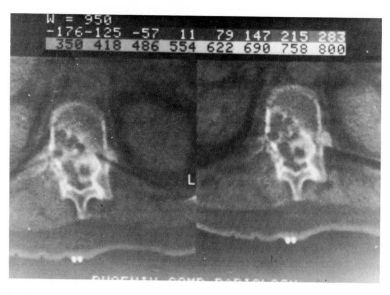

FIG. 20. CT axial sections from adjacent levels of thoracic spine following placement of intrathecal metrizamide. Note that bone destruction from the breast metastasis involves the vertebra and the right side of the neural arch extending into the paraspinal musculature. Also, notice deviation of the spinal cord to the left from the epidural mass effect. No cord invasion is present.

ning). Developed as a clinically usable tool by Ambrose and Houusfield for head scanning in 1973 (1,20), it immediately revolutionized neuroradiographic imaging. Shortly after, further developments, which include the use of multiple photomultiplier tubes as radiation detectors and computer modifications, thus allowing reconstruction of the axial image, made body scanning possible. As newer generation scanners became available, refinements in software reconstructions, fast high resolution scanning, thin overlapping sections, and meticulous attention to detail have provided the clinician with a noninvasive method of examining the spinal cord and surrounding structures. The ability to vary the window width and center allow all structures from dense bone to more lucent fat to be examined individually or together. The multiplanar reconstruction capability allows saggital, coronal, oblique, and more recently 3-dimensional visualization from the initial axial section (16). This is a function of the computer and produces no additional radiation or delay of examination to the patient.

Figure 19 shows an axial and reconstructed coronal section through the spine of an 18-month-old child found to have a L3-4 spine infection but unexplained left leg pain. The vertebral body infection is clearly demonstrated along with the left psoas abscess as a low density area in the muscle and vertebral body. Appropriate antibiotics and immobilization cleared the infection, and on a subsequent scan, sclerosis of the vertebra and resolution of the psoas abscess were found. The entire diagnosis was made without any invasive procedures, although biopsy and aspiration

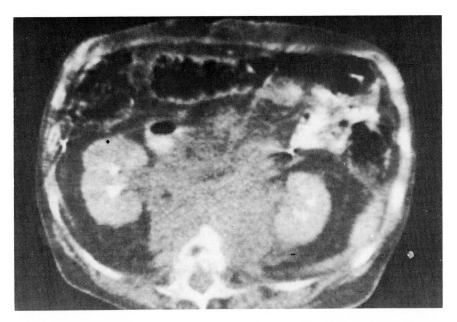

FIG. 21. CT axial section of mid-abdomen showing extensive pancreatic tumor mass that invades the retroperitoneum, displacing kidneys laterally and invading vertebral body.

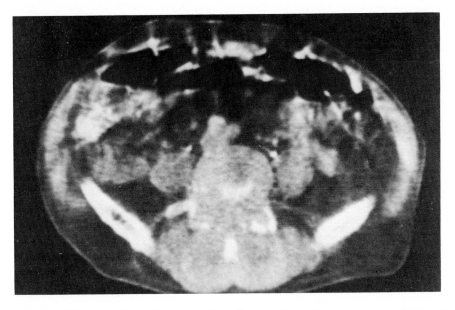

FIG. 22. CT axial section of lumbosacral junction showing replacement of normal bone by tumors from metastatic renal clear cell carcinoma. This is the same patient as in Figures 17 and 18.

of the abscess could easily have been done with CT guidance. Radiation exposure was limited by using only a few thin columnated slices.

Figure 20 shows the metastatic involvement of a thoracic vertebra, epidural space, and paraspinal region in a 70-year-old female with known breast cancer. She presented with radicular pain not clearly apparent on myelography, which demonstrated a minimal extradural compression without block, similarly seen on this CT section. Delineation of the paraspinal involvement, which was not diagnosed by other studies, explains the focal nerve root involvement. This is an example of how CT is used to supplement an equivocal metrizamide myelogram. The scans may be done immediately or within 3 to 4 hours of the myelogram without loss of information.

CT may also reveal occult retroperitoneal or pelvic mass as the cause of back pain. This is seen in Fig. 21, where a pancreatic carcinoma has invaded the entire retroperitoneum and bony vertebra. Figure 22 shows the extensive bony destruction and nerve entrapment in a patient with metastatic renal carcinoma. This was the same patient in whom arterial embolization was discussed above.

Spinal stenosis from bony hypertrophy, congenital scarring, or masses are clearly demonstrated. The left half of Fig. 23 shows a disk herniation into the canal and extending into the right lateral recess. For comparison, the outline of a normal round subarachnoid space and nerve roots, seen from the level above, are shown on the right.

This disk was seen without the use of contrast and was surgically excised. Several papers describe the technique required for adequate visualization of herniated disks (7,16,28,43).

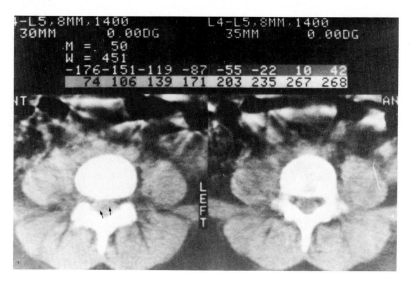

FIG. 23. CT axial sections through L4–5 on the left and L3–4 on the right. Note kidney-bean shaped disk in the canal (↑) compressing the subarachnoid space. Compare this with the normal round configuration at the level above.

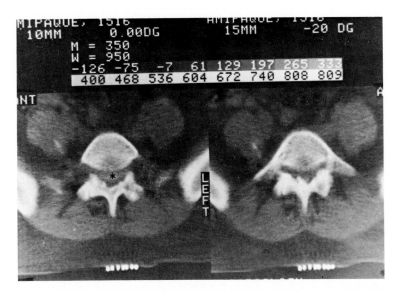

FIG. 24. CT axial sections at L5–S1 on the left and L5 on the right. Note the higher density semilunar disk (*) obstructing the spinal canal. L5 level also shows a narrowed bony spinal canal.

The utilization of CT to visualize herniated disks may prove to be one of its most valuable uses. As spatial and contrast resolution continue to improve, there will be a concomitant decrease in the need of the invasive procedures mentioned above to diagnose disk disease. Just as important is the ability to rule this entity out reliably. The role of CT in evaluating the postoperative back should also expand as studies show that the more invasive procedures are reliably replaced.

Various measurements of the bony canal are possible, including those calculated by computer. Done at specific center and window settings, the measurements may be compared with charts showing AP, interpedicular, and square area for each spinal level (22,40). These findings are enhanced by planes reconstructed for neural foramina evaluation when abnormal spinal curves or fractures are present that would prevent the obtaining of axial slices parallel to the vertebral body. This relationship is important for accurate measurement of the spinal canal.

Figure 24 shows a complete block at the L5-S1 level from a large disk that has herniated into the canal. This finding was subsequently supported by metrizamide myelography (Fig. 25) and confirmed at surgery.

Figure 26 demonstrates lateral recess compromise on the right L4-5 level. Here again CT supplementation of the myelogram was useful. This compromise generally results from encroachment into the foramina from the superior facet of the vertebra below.

Unrecognized spinal stenosis, located either in the central or in the lateral recess, is an important cause of failed back surgery syndrome where pain is the primary symptom.

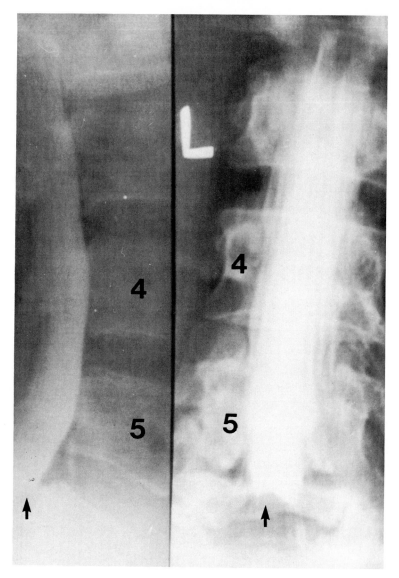

FIG. 25. Metrizamide myelogram of patient in Fig. 24. This shows complete obstruction from herniation of the entire L5–S1 disk material into the spinal canal.

The appearance of arachnoiditis with distortion of the subarachnoid pouch is clearly shown with the axial view on CT and differentiates the defect from bony causes. Defects from arachnoiditis in the postoperative back are at times difficult to distinguish from associated facet hypertrophy, callus formation from fusion, or recurrent disk. CT clearly allows this separation to be made, as seen in Fig. 27. Here a combination of arachnoiditis and facet hypertrophy form the etiology of this

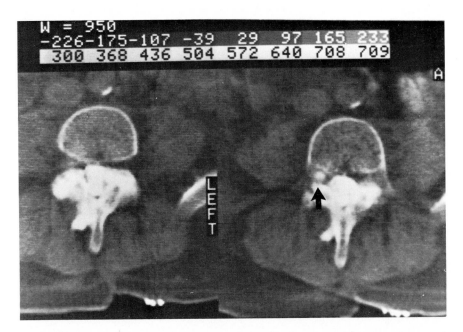

FIG. 26. CT axial sections through adjacent L4–5 sections showing distortion of the metrizamide filled subarachnoid space, marked hypertrophy of the facet joints, and loss of right lateral recess (↑) with superior facet from below encroaching into this space.

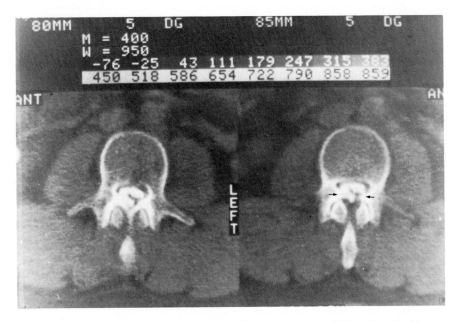

FIG. 27. CT axial sections from adjacent L3 cuts showing distortion of the subarachnoid space from arachnoiditis and bony spur from the medial facet joints. These could not be appreciated on plain films.

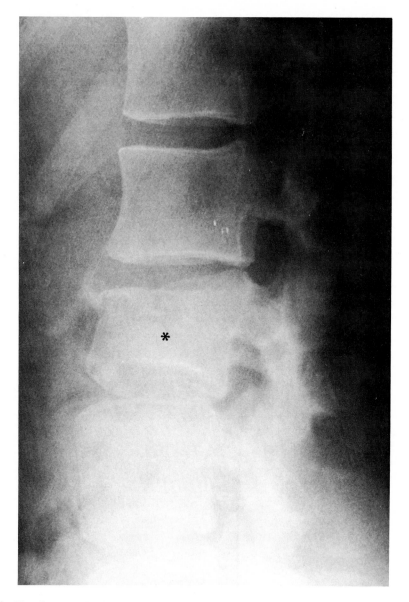

FIG. 28. Compression fracture of the lumbar vertebra with loss of height. No evidence of bone in the spinal canal or posterior neural arch.

patient's back pain, which developed several years after the initial surgery. Note distortion of the metrizamide-filled subarachnoid space and encroaching facet tips from the medial aspect.

Evaluation of vertebral fractures or penetrating missile injuries has been remarkably improved with CT. Figures 28 and 29 are examples of how plain films

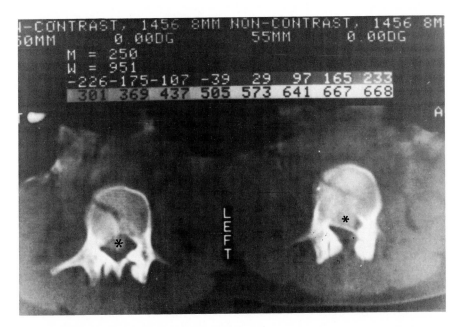

FIG. 29. CT axial sections showing oblique fracture line through vertebral body and left lamina. Also note the large fragment (*) comprising the spinal canal.

demonstrate loss of vertical height but poorly show the contents of the spinal canal and neural arch. On the CT section, note the large fragment that extends into the canal. This is not seen on the standard lateral view, shown for comparison.

Conventional tomography may be used, but AP and lateral projections have been estimated to yield approximately ten times the radiation dose of a comparable CT study. The lack of need to move or turn the patient and the ability to scan through orthopedic devices are additional advantages.

The limitation of CT in trauma is the poor evaluation of vertical height with axial projections. This disadvantage is lessened by reconstructed images but that image remains inferior to standard projections. At this time, it is suggested that antero-posterior and lateral roentgenographs followed by CT be used to evaluate the traumatized spine.

SUMMARY

One can easily be confused by the numerous diagnostic modalities available since the addition of several new procedures, as defined in the text, unless careful consideration is given to the patient's findings and an orderly process for confirming those findings is adhered to.

This presentation has suggested a plan for implementing the various tools, along with a brief discussion and case examples, that demonstrate the value of each. The reader is referred to the numerous excellent papers that discuss the various areas in greater depth.

As with all new discoveries in the medical field, CT will need close evaluation for its ultimate role in low back pain and sciatica. Prospective studies will be needed to determine the incidence of asymptomatic spinal stenosis, herniated or bulging intervertebral disk, lateral recess compromise, and facet joint abnormalities as seen by CT, since improving technology continually allows more detailed and definitive visualization of the back. It will be necessary to correlate these anatomical findings with specific signs and symptoms so that unnecessary and unreliable examinations can be eliminated.

REFERENCES

1. Ambrose, J. (1973): Computerized transverse scanning (tomography). Part 2: Clinical application. *Br. J. Radiol.*, 46:1023–1047.
2. Antoku, S., and Russell, W. J. (1971): Dose to the active bone marrow, gonads, and skin from roentgenography and fluoroscopy. *Radiology*, 101:669–678.
3. Ardran, G. M., and Crooks, H. E. (1957): Gonad radiation dose from diagnostic procedures. *Br. J. Radiol.*, 30:295–297.
4. Arnell, S., and Lidström, F. (1931): Myelography with Skiodan (Abrodil). *Acta Radiol.*, 12:287–288.
5. Brodsky, A. E., and Binder, W. F. (1979): Lumbar Discography. *Spine*, 4:110–120.
6. Burton, C. V. (1978): Lumbosacral arachnoiditis. *Spine*, 3:24–30.
7. Carrera, G. F., Williams, A. L., and Haughton, V. M. (1980): Computed tomography in sciatica. *Radiology*, 137:433–437.
8. Colonna, P. C., and Friedenberg, Z. B. (1949): The disc syndrome: Results of the conservative care of patients with positive myelograms. *J. Bone Joint Surg.*, 31:614–618.
9. Dandy, W. E. (1919): Roentgenography of the brain after the injection of air into the spinal canal. *Ann. Surg.*, 70:397–403.
10. Dandy, W. E. (1941): Ventriculography following the injection of air into the cerebral ventricles. *Ann. Surg.*, 68:5–11.
11. Eisenberg, R. L., Akin, J. R., Hedgcock, M. W. (1979): Single, well centered lateral view of lumbosacral spine: is coned view necessary? *Am. J. Roentgenol.*, 133:711–713.
12. Forrester, D. M., and Brown, J. C. (1980): Radiographic Evaluation of Back Pain. *Contemporary Diagnostic Radiology*, No. 6: 1–5, The Williams & Wilkins Co., Baltimore, Maryland.
13. Friedenberg, Z. B., and Shoemaker, R. C. (1954): The results of nonoperative treatment of ruptured lumbar discs. *Amer. J. Surg.*, 88:933–935.
14. Fullenlove, T. M., and Williams, A. J. (1957): Comparative roentgen findings in symptomatic and asymptomatic backs. *Radiology*, 68:572–574.
15. Gargano, F. P., Meyer, J. D., and Sheldon, J. J. (1974): Transfemoral ascending lumbar catheterization of the epidural veins in lumbar disc disease. Clinical application and results in the diagnosis of the herniated intervertebral disc of the lumbar spine. *Radiology*, 111:329–336.
16. Glenn, W. V., Jr., Rhodes, M. L., Altschuler, E. M., Wiltse, L. L., Kostanek, C., and Kuo, Y. M. (1979): Multiplanar display computerized body tomography application in the lumbar spine. *Spine*, 4:382–392.
17. Hall, F. M. (1976): Overutilization of radiological examinations. Opinion. *Radiology*, 120:443–448.
18. Holmes, H. E., and Rothman, R. H. (1976): The Pennsylvania Plan: An algorithm for the management of lumbar degenerative disc disease. *Spine*, 4:156–167.
19. Holt, E. P., Jr. (1968): The question of discography. *J. Bone Joint Surg.*, 50A: 720–725.
20. Houusfield, G. N. (1973): Computerized transverse axial scanning (tomography). Part 1: Description of system. *Br. J. Radiol.*, 46:1016–1022.
21. Kirkaldy-Willis, W. H. (1979): A more precise diagnosis for low-back pain. *Spine*, 4:102–109.
22. Lee, B. C. P., Kazam, E., Newman, A. D. (1978): Computed tomography of the spine and spinal cord. *Radiology*, 128:95–102.
23. Lewit, K., Sereghy, T. (1975): Lumbar peridurography with special regard to the anatomy of the lumbar peridural space. *Neuroradiology*, 8:233–240.

24. Lindblom, K. (1948): Diagnostic puncture of intervertebral discs in sciatica. *Acta. Orthop. Scand.*, 17:231–239.
25. Luyendijk, W. (1963): Canalography, roentgenological examination of the peridural space in the lumbosacral part of the vertebral canal. *J. Belge Radiol.*, 46:236–253.
26. MacNab, I. (1971): Negative disc explorations. *J. Bone Joint Surg.*, 53A:891–903.
27. McRae, D. (1955): Asymptomatic intervertebral disc protrusion. *Acta Radiol.*, 46:9–27.
28. Meyer, G. A., Haughton, V. M., and Williams, A. L. (1979): Diagnosis of herniated lumbar disc with computed tomography. *N. Engl. J. Med.*, 301:1166–1167.
29. Mixter, W. J., and Barr, J. S. (1934): Rupture of the intervertebral disc with involvement of the spinal canal. *N. Engl. J. Med.*, 112:210.
30. Nachemson, A. L. (1976): The lumbar spine: An Orthopaedic Challenge. *Spine*, 1:59–71.
31. Rhea, J. T., De Luca, S. A., Llewellyn, H. J., and Boyd, R. J. (1980): The oblique view: an unnecessary component of the initial adult lumbar spine examination. *Radiology*, 134:45–47.
32. Roberson, G. H., Hatten, H. P., and Hesselink, J. H. (1979): Epidurography: Selective catheter technique and review of 53 cases. *Am. J. Roentgenol.*, 132:787–793.
33. Roberts, F. F., Kishore, P. R. S., and Cunningham, M. E. (1978): Routine oblique radiography of the pediatric lumbar spine: is it necessary? *Am. J. Roentgenol.*, 131:297–298.
34. Sachett, J. F., and Strother, C. M. (1980): *New Techniques in Myelography*, Harper and Row Publishers, Inc., Philadelphia, Pennsylvania.
35. Sanford, H., and Doub, H. P. (1941): Epidurography, a method of roentgenologic visualization of protruded intervertebral discs. *Radiology*, 36:712–716.
36. Shleien, B., Tucker, T. T., and Johnson, D. W. (1979): The mean active bone marrow dose to the adult population of the United States from diagnostic radiology. DHEW Publ (FDA) 77-8013. U.S. Govt. Print. Office, Washington, D.C.
37. Spengler, D. M., and Freeman, C. W. (1979): Patient selection for lumbar discectomy. *Spine*, 4:129–134.
38. Splithoff, C. A. (1953): Lumbosacral junction. Roentgenographic comparison of the patients with and without backaches. *JAMA*, 152:1610–1613.
39. Torgerson, W. R., and Dotter, W. E. (1976): Comparative roentgenographic study of the asymptomatic and symptomatic lumbar spine. *J. Bone Joint Surg.*, 58A:850–853.
40. Ullrich, C. G., and Kieffer, S. A. (1980): Computed tomographic evaluation of the lumbar spine: Quantitative aspects and sagittalcoronal reconstruction. In: *Radiographic Evaluation of the Spine*, edited by M. J. D. Post, pp. 88–107. Masson Publishing U. S. A., Inc., New York.
41. Van Damme, W., Hessels, G., Verhelst, M., Van Laer, L., and Van Es, I. (1979): Relative efficacy of clinical examination, electromyography, plain film radiography, myelography and lumbar phlebography in the diagnosis of low back pain and sciatica. *Neuroradiology*, 18:109–118.
42. Webster, E. W., and Merrill, O. E. (1957): Radiation hazards, II Measurements of gonadal dose in radiographic examination. *N. Engl. J. Med.*, 257:811–819.
43. Williams, A. L., Haughton, V. M., and Syvertsen, A. (1980): Computed tomography in the diagnosis of herniated nucleus pulposus. *Radiology*, 135:95–99.
44. Wise, R. E., and Weiford, E. C. (1951): X-ray visualization of intervertebral disc: Report of case. *Cleve. Clin. Q.*, 18:127–130.

Chronic Low Back Pain, edited by
M. Stanton-Hicks and Robert Boas.
Raven Press, New York © 1982.

A Cognitive-Behavioral Perspective in the Assessment and Treatment of Chronic Low Back Pain

Lawrence E. Peterson

Pain Control Unit, University of Massachusetts Medical Center and Department of Psychology, Worcester State Hospital, Worcester, Massachusetts 01605

The past 20 years have produced a dramatic increase in the variety of psychological assessment and treatment interventions in chronic low back pain. The purpose of this chapter is to describe a cognitive-behavioral approach to psychological evaluation and treatment. The procedures are designed to be incorporated into a multidisciplinary team approach to chronic low back pain and complement thorough physical and medical examinations and treatments. The material that will be presented below is clinical in nature, rather than a review of the literature.

Traditionally, a disease model has provided the major conceptual framework for understanding pain. The shortcomings of this model and a more useful schema are presented by Loeser elsewhere in this volume. Loeser's definitions of nociception, pain, suffering, and pain behavior (13) will be followed in the discussion below.

PSYCHOLOGICAL EVALUATION

Historically, psychological or psychiatric evaluation of a chronic back pain problem was directed at a request for a differential diagnosis among four main alternatives: (a) hysterical neurosis (a conversion reaction); (b) a psychophysiological disorder, musculoskeletal type (presumably mediated via the autonomic nervous system); (c) malingering; and (d) a neurological disorder. Diagnoses appropriate to these alternatives are contained in the *Diagnostic and Statistical Manual of Mental Disorders* of the American Psychiatric Association (1,2). The core of the referral seemed to be, "Is this pain psychogenic?" Patients seemed to perceive that question as, "Is this pain imaginary?"

This approach to evaluation has proved to be exceptionally difficult and often unrewarding. Part of this may be due to reliability problems with the category system, problems that may be alleviated by the newest edition of the manual (2). However, it seems more likely that the difficulty arises from asking the wrong question, "Does chronic low back pain have a psychological or a physical etiology?" For most cases, perhaps all, both seem to be involved.

Finally, a logical problem occurs when inferences about "psychogenic" factors are made simply on the absence of physical findings. No one can prove that something, in this case a physical cause, does not exist, as patients repeatedly point out. Thus, in a psychological evaluation, it is necessary to seek positive indications of the importance of factors such as stress or conditioning.

In this regard, Fordyce (12) has demonstrated the importance of operant conditioning processes in the total pain problem, specifically focusing on pain behavior. There is abundant evidence that responses followed by reinforcement are more likely to recur. Both the addition of a desirable stimulus (positive reinforcement) and the removal of a negative one (negative reinforcement) in a contingent fashion increases the probability that the response will be repeated. Sternbach (25), on the other hand, points to the importance of interpersonal factors ("games") and to the debilitating effects of chronic pain, especially the production of depression.

The assessment procedure presented below takes a broad focus in order to obtain information on the patient's pain, suffering, and pain behaviors without attempting to assign primary importance to any area. Evaluation of nociception is beyond the scope of psychological assessment. In each aspect of the pain problem the patient's thoughts, feelings, and behaviors are specifically sought.

The evaluation is designed to be done on an outpatient basis. The main objective is to understand the back pain problem in the context of the individual's total functioning. This is facilitated by having the person maintain his/her typical schedule. The core evaluation consists of two parts. First, each patient is asked to complete at home two written tests, a Minnesota Multiphasic Personality Inventory (MMPI), and a Daily Activity Schedule. The MMPI is an empirically based personality test that gives important clues as to the person's psychological functioning (10). Second, patients come to the clinic for a structured interview. Whenever possible, significant family members are also seen (23).

MMPI

Because of its frequent use in psychological evaluations in the clinical setting and its frequent inclusion in research projects on chronic back pain, a brief description of the MMPI is in order. The test can be taken by anyone who is over 16 years of age with a sixth grade reading level in English. The person marks an answer sheet "True" or "False" for each of 566 items. It usually takes the patient between 1 and 2 hr to complete and can be scored in approximately 15 min.

The basic test profile consists of three validity scales and 10 clinical scales arranged on a profile sheet. Each scale has a mean of 50 and a standard deviation of 10. There are also 41 critical items that can be followed up in the interview when they are checked off in the keyed direction. Included are items that may indicate serious disturbance of cognitive function or behavior.

Two types of MMPI interpretation are prevalent. The first approach tries to describe the personality characteristics of a particular patient or of patients with chronic back pain in general. Here, it is the person who is labeled. This approach is not particularly helpful in understanding the individual patient or in predicting treatment outcomes (5,9,18,28). The second approach utilizes the MMPI to indicate the likelihood of certain thoughts, feelings, and behaviors that have particular relevance to pain. Here, it is the problems that are labeled and the response probabilities that are described. For example, how likely is the person to experience bodily distress and to complain about it? How aversive or reinforcing are increases in activity likely to be? Is the person likely to be receptive to explanations of his/her pain that include non-somatic factors?

The response-probability approach requires that the test data be interpreted in the context of other information. Of particular interest is the overall level of distress, the presence and severity of depression, and the responses on the critical items. The MMPI is not used to differentiate "organic" from "functional" cases, to make a psychiatric diagnosis, or to predict success in treatment. As noted, the literature is equivocal regarding the ability of the test to do any of these in randomized group studies and post hoc comparisons. It is not justified in the individual clinical evaluation.

In the interpretation of MMPI scale scores, the norms on Minnesota "normals" may be inappropriate as the comparison group (10). Many pain clinics compute norms for their own population and consider the data in this light as well. Prior to evaluating the tests, it is also helpful to find out the medications (and their dosages) being taken by patients.

Daily Activity Schedule

Also completed before the interview is a Daily Activity Schedule covering a 7-day period. This form makes an hourly record of all the patient's activities for the week. Patients simply check a key for the numbers representing the activities engaged in and enter the numbers on a record form. This provides a general guide to "downtime", level of social contact, and a picture of the daily routine.

The Interview

The second part of the evaluation is a structured interview conducted with the patient after reviewing the other materials. It requires approximately 1½ hr. Establishing rapport can be difficult since patients often see the purpose of the psychological evaluation as proving that they are "crazy" and the pain is "all in their head," an opinion that they may believe their physicians have had for some time. In general, most become cooperative and accept the possibility that stress or conditioning plays a role in their pain.

The interview begins with a review of the pain problem, its history, description, and location. Patients are asked to rate the severity or intensity of their pain on a 0 to 100 scale. Included is a rating of their average pain, their worst pain, and their pain at the time of the interview. Also, what is the daily pattern? Morning, afternoon, and evening ratings are requested.

Next is a thorough review of factors that exacerbate or diminish the pain and the sequence of events. Often patients describe a pattern of engaging in physical activity until pain occurs, then resting. What is the schedule of analgesic medication? As Fordyce (12) has cogently pointed out, "as needed" medication would be the strategy employed by a learning psychologist to condition in strong behavior. Specifically, pain behaviors are reinforced by a powerful reward, often a narcotic.

The role of stress, the level of tension and anxiety present, and the person's view of these processes is explored. Is the pain a stressor generating a substantial autonomic/endocrine response? When the pain is severe, what is the mood? Fear, anger, frustration, depression? Most patients report that anxiety and pain have a mutually enhancing effect and that pain can be magnified by thinking about it too much. Is there a pattern of poor stress coping? How is the pain related to other stresses?

Attention is focused on the average day in the recent past and the Daily Activity Schedule is reviewed with the patient. How does the pain affect the daily schedule? The following areas are specifically investigated: sleep, sexual activities, family, employment, hobbies, and household chores. What is the gain, loss, or change in these areas?

How is the patient coping with the chronic pain? Some psychologists believe that depression is a nearly universal consequence of chronic pain. If there are indications of depression, the area is thoroughly explored using the Hamilton Rating Scale for Depression. An important question is the likelihood of suicide. Does the person have adequate coping strategies? Addiction to narcotic medication complicates the situation and adds to the risk. The same is true of alcohol.

A related problem is anger and its control. Does the patient withdraw, yell, hit? In exploring these affective areas, the patient's cognitions can be elicited too. What does he/she think causes the pain? How can it be controlled? Eliminated? Does the patient view his/her role as active or passive? Has the patient had previous psychiatric intervention?

The last portion of the interview is a brief trial of relaxation and imagery tasks. First, an inquiry is made into any experiences or training that the patient may have had in muscle relaxation, meditation, hypnosis, or biofeedback. Then using a comfortable reclining chair, the patient is given some brief muscle-relaxation instruction. In addition, some trials are made with visual images such as a beach or meadow. Depending on the interest of the patient, brief trials with electromyographic or finger temperature biofeedback may be given.

This type of psychological evaluation and the treatment recommendations that are derived from it can be illustrated most clearly by a case example. It is representative of a "difficult" patient referred for evaluation and has been disguised to protect the identity of the client. Only summary information will be presented in each section.

Case of Ms. X

Ms. X, an outpatient, is a 50-year-old married female referred for psychological evaluation in regard to her chronic low back pain. She completed an MMPI and Daily Activity Schedule and was seen for interview alone and with her husband.

History of the problem. Ms. X has a 10-year history of the current pain in her back. It began after a fall when she slipped and landed hard on the base of her spine. Within 2 years she has had five hospitalizations, including three surgical procedures: a lower lumbar fusion, a coccygectomy, and a repeat lumbar fusion. Pain persisted and an extensive work-up was completed at a Boston hospital. No further positive findings were reported. Her medication at the time of the interview included Percodan p.r.n. (or 5–6/day), Valium (diazepam) p.r.n., and Mylanta.

Other medical history. The patient has had nine other surgical procedures, mild backache and migraine since adolescence, and considerable digestive distress. She is now being treated for a duodenal ulcer.

Family history. Ms. X is the older of two daughters; both parents are deceased. She is a high school graduate who worked until her marriage. She currently lives with her husband, a second-shift foreman in a manufacturing plant. They have three grown children who have all married and moved away from the area.

Observations. She is a heavy-set woman, brought to the interview in a wheelchair by her husband. The patient's response to the MMPI and a psychological evaluation was quite negative. She described the test as "demeaning" and stated clearly that the pain was in her back, not in her head. She objected that she was "not crazy" and was angry at being "given the run-around" by the "doctors." There was a pervasive attitude of resentment and criticism of her treatment. She expressed discouragement, especially at being such a burden to her husband. As the interview progressed, she became more cooperative and, in fact, wanted to have a lengthy discussion on hypnosis at the conclusion.

Pain description. The pain was described as constant, dull, and non-throbbing pain in the lower back, mostly on the right side. It did not radiate into the legs. On a 0 to 100 subjective scale, she rated her average pain as 90 with a range of 60 to 100. It was worse in the morning. Movement sometimes preceded sharp, grabbing pains. She described her mood as "frustrated" and said that she occasionally gets depressed and wishes she were dead. However, she denied ever having suicidal ideation and has never had psychiatric treatment. She stated that stress "has nothing to do with the pain."

Factors exacerbating and diminishing the pain. Virtually all physical activities exacerbate the pain, particularly bending, walking, sitting, riding in the car, and standing. Weather and stress are unrelated. Factors that diminish the pain include bed, Percodan, and "distracting myself by reading."

Daily activities. Ms. X has over 23 hr/day of downtime, spending virtually all her time in bed or in the wheelchair. She does some cooking and occasionally goes out to visit friends. Her husband waits on her and appears extremely solicitous. She reports that he is "too good to me." She sleeps only 4 hr each night, which she attributes to pain interference and not feeling tired. She has gained over 35 lb in the past 4 years. Sexual activity is absent. Her hobbies include reading, keeping up with current events, and crocheting.

Coping with the pain. Ms. X copes poorly with the pain. She sometimes takes extra medication, feels irritable and resentful, and has virtually stopped her former daily routine. Her MMPI is valid and not elevated out of the normal range. It is very guarded. Women with similar profiles would be described as likely to have somatic complaints, unlikely to express any psychological problem or be reinforced by activity, and likely to have a fairly stereotypic, traditional view of a woman's role. Inactivity and isolation from people are frequent. Her Hamilton Rating for Depression was moderate and largely composed of the somatic items.

Relaxation and imagery. On simple tasks of relaxation and visual imagery, she did well, showing good concentration, vivid visual imagery, and enthusiasm for the task.

Other evaluations. All physical and X-ray findings, and diagnostic test results were negative. Physical therapy evaluation showed significant muscular weakness, and a substantial amount of grimacing, complaining, and groaning was noted.

What analysis and treatment recommendations can be generated from these data? It seems probable that much of Ms. X's behavioral, cognitive, and affective response systems are influenced by her pain and in return have become contributors to the overall pain response. Virtually all of her daily behaviors related directly to pain. She has restricted her physical activity almost totally, schedules her few activities around her Percodan schedule, is dependent on her husband for the basic necessities of daily living. Regardless of the original nociceptive component of her pain, her current pain behaviors are being consistently reinforced by her medication and her husband's attention.

Her cognitive functions are not grossly impaired. However, her cognitive style is rigid, sour, and pessimistic, and the possibility of thinking about her pain from any but a physical perspective seems remote. Helpless, hopeless sentences prevail, and she occasionally admits to depression. Her general affective experience is largely unpleasant, with anger, tension, and sadness prevailing. There is substantial suffering.

On the more positive side, she responded well and enjoyed the relaxation and imagery tasks. She was interested in mental "games," smiled, and followed directions well. There is also some indication from this that interpersonal contact may be more rewarding than the other material indicates.

A supportive, multifaceted treatment approach seems called for in this case. Many would suggest beginning with detoxification from the Percodan, at least putting it on a regular interval schedule. A major component would be a physical therapy program utilizing exercises, eventually walking, and increased participation in normal daily activities. These tasks would have to be designed to exercise criteria, not to pain, and would include her husband. A supportive multifaceted patient education program is required to provide her with a more adaptive psychophysiological model of pain. Finally, some analgesic medication or blocks would be included.

The literature is far from clear on whether or not such a program would succeed. Inpatient multidisciplinary approaches such as this seem to produce success rates of 30 to 60% (12,25,26). Predicting Ms. X's specific response beyond base rates such as this is not possible. Increased activity and reduced narcotic medication can be seen as likely while treatment is taking place. Long-term substantial reduction in subjective pain report in cases with a poor premorbid history is less likely (17). Outpatient status throughout treatment in a case like this occurs infrequently in the literature. A complicating factor in predicting outcome from psychological evaluations is the lack of agreement on what constitutes success.

A final major role of the psychologist and the psychological evaluation is to guard against hasty or unwarranted use of labels such as "psychogenic." To return to the referral question, "Is the pain psychogenic?" The present view is that all chronic pain is influenced by psychological factors and that chronic pain also has its own debilitating psychological effects. Any "either/or" construction of the problem seems too narrow. Similarly, it appears that any comprehensive treatment program for chronic back pain must include psychological components.

COGNITIVE-BEHAVIORAL TREATMENT STRATEGIES

The most prevalent form of psychological intervention with people who have problems is individual counseling or psychotherapy. This is typically done on an outpatient basis, follows one of several well-defined theoretical models (e.g., psychoanalytic, Rogerian), and has shown limited success with chronic back pain. More and more, clinics and multidisciplinary teams are incorporating a wide range of psychological interventions (4,11,14,26). These include operant conditioning, a variety of group therapy programs, stress management training—including muscle relaxation and biofeedback—and cognitive-behavioral programs such as stress innoculation, guided imagery, and self-hypnosis.

The first widely used psychologically based adjunctive treatment was operant conditioning, directed at modifying the patient's pain behaviors. Fordyce (12,13) has been the principal proponent of this approach, drawing heavily on the work of Skinner (24). Operant conditioning procedures are designed to decrease the frequency of pain behavior and increase the frequency of well behavior. The general paradigm is to arrange the contingencies to reinforce well behavior and to ignore and not reinforce pain behavior. These operant conditioning strategies make up a portion of the cognitive-behavioral approach.

The Development of Cognitive-Behavioral Management

The operant and classical conditioning approaches have been expanded in the field of behavior therapy to incorporate thinking and other cognitive functions. The specific application of cognitive-behavioral approaches in chronic pain has been described by Bresler (6,7), DeGood (11), and Meichenbaum (19), and was recently reviewed by Turk and Genest (27). The basic thrust of the cognitive strategies has been to encourage new ways of perceiving and thinking about nociceptive stimuli and to devise coping strategies. In redirecting the perception of the client, some of the procedures have been borrowed from hypnosis, particularly the works of Hilgard (15) and Orne (21).

The cognitive-behavioral approach attempts to assist the client in ameliorating the problem at the level of perception (pain), suffering, and pain behavior. Nociceptive stimuli are not addressed directly. To the extent that nociceptive input is a significant part of the problem, the cognitive-behavioral approach is adjunctive and will not solve the problem. The patient may learn to cope better, but other therapeutic efforts must be successful for complete relief. On the other hand, the nociceptive stimuli may have ceased, and thus relief is a possibility with cognitive-behavioral approaches.

Cognitive-Behavioral Contributions in a Multidisciplinary Setting

Consultation

A cognitive-behavioral analysis may generate useful ideas for the implementation of other treatment strategies. For example, in most cases p.r.n. medication regimes of narcotics can be replaced by regular interval regimes, even when the medication is to be retained in the overall treatment plan. Similarly, exercise programs can be utilized in which the patient works to a criterion (e.g., 5 repetitions or 200 yards) rather than to pain tolerance. Indeed, many of these ideas now have general acceptance.

Patient Education

A second role for a cognitive-behavioral approach is in patient education. Despite hours with medical personnel, most patients seem to have a very unsophisticated model of pain from a psychophysiological perspective. To many, it is the simple "either/or" two-category system of diagnosis, that is, either "It's in my back and can be repaired," or "It's in my head, and I'm crazy." The subjectively compelling experience of pain as located in the back causes patients to reject this latter view.

However, most patients also acknowledge that stress seems to magnify pain or that a fascinating book provides complete, albeit temporary, distraction. How can this be explained? Since it has been helpful with non-pain problems, a counseling model developed with another psychologist, Paul Gerson, has been utilized as a framework for teaching patients a more complex psychophysiological model (21).

Brief or more extended lectures are given to patients and can be part of assessment, individual treatment, or group treatment. The purpose of the lectures is to enlist the patient's active participation and to share a new model of pain.

The core of the system is to describe a person as a triangle with three key reacting systems—a cognitive system, an affective system, and a behavioral system—for clarity in communicating thoughts, feelings, and behaviors. Thoughts include remembering, imagining, planning, and perception—activities that go on in one's head. Feelings are moods such as anger, fear, and sadness, and describe body states. Fear, for example, has often been related to adrenalin. Finally, behaviors are what the person does, such as walking and talking. Where does pain fit? Patients usually perceive quickly that all systems are involved. Each patient seems to have his/her own combination. Loeser's diagram can be drawn in addition to the triangle to illustrate this interrelationship (13). This "triangle" model takes little time to present and serves as a simple descriptive tool.

What are stress and tension, and what role do they play in pain? Most clients are conceptually unsophisticated but still nod vigorously when a "vicious cycle" of pain leading to adrenalin/nonadrenalin leading to worse pain is described. Further, it seems obvious to most of them that if they could be calm and relaxed, the pain would "hurt" less.

The "sabertooth tiger lecture" illustrates a conditioned fear response. Confrontation with a sabertooth tiger by our ancestors involved a strong, automatic fight-or-flight response mediated by autonomic/endocrine responses. Those who failed did not continue in the gene pool. Unfortunately for our patients, the danger signal that turns on the system is their pain. The short-term consequences are anxiety, irritability, and so on. A long-term consequence may be depression. Certainly there is ample evidence that depression is a frequent component in the individual with chronic pain.

Cognitive-Behavioral Pain Management

Finally, a cognitive-behavioral approach can generate direct treatment. In order to monitor the desired changes in the thoughts, feelings, and behaviors, a baseline is necessary. One of the core ingredients of this treatment approach is collecting data, typically in a behavioral journal. The first step in treatment involves collecting baseline data and defining the treatment goals. Although data from sources other than the client are useful, primary data collection responsibility falls to the client. The program is individualized, but all patients keep track of all medication, physical activities (both type and amount), and subjective pain at least once each hour. Except when medical or surgical treatment or detoxification requires hospitalization, the patient remains in his/her home environment. It should be stressed that the cognitive and behavioral interventions are carried out in conjunction with other aspects of treatment such as physical and occupational therapy.

While the baseline is being established, treatment goals are negotiated and ranked as to importance and contrasted with problems. Problems here are defined as those thoughts, feelings, and behaviors that the client has but does not want. Goals are thoughts, feelings, and behaviors that the client wants but does not have. The point of treatment is for patients to achieve positive goals, not to eliminate problems. For example, learning to be calm and relaxed, rather than stopping anxiety, is the goal-oriented approach. The advantage of this is highlighted in the interpersonal behavior area. Thus, abstaining from such behavior as arguing, withdrawing, or fighting leaves unspecified what is to happen. Talking calmly, remaining with people, and going out for a nice meal specify the goals.

The final treatment contract includes the means that will be employed to achieve the goals. Most involve some strategy for coping with pain by acquiring skills in relaxation, cognitive restructuring, or contingency management. Immediate mastery of pain or its elimination is considered an unlikely outcome. Coping better, handling anxiety and depression, and adapting to necessary restrictions in occupation or activity are suggested as more realistic. For example, for many patients with chronic back pain, employment prospects may be almost nil because such patients are considered high risks.

Some form of relaxation training is usually carried out. As in the overall analysis, the problem of anxiety and tension is considered from cognitive, affective, and behavioral perspectives. Cognitive elements include worry, specific fears, difficulty in concentrating, and beliefs that something awful is going to happen. Affective aspects are from autonomic and endocrine arousal: butterflies in the stomach, sweaty palms, fear, and so on. Typical behavior includes restlessness, pacing, and nail biting.

Individuals have different patterns of anxiety with varying contributions in each area. Different procedures for teaching relaxation are more directed to one system than another. Cognitive changes are the focus in the autogenic training of Schultz and Luthe (22), meditation, and the training of Benson (3). These procedures involve practicing relaxing sentences, eliminating distracting thoughts, and concentrating on warm relaxed heavy pleasant sensations in the body.

Direct intervention in the autonomic/endocrine arousal response is illustrated by the work on biofeedback and the tension/release muscle relaxation training of Jacobson (16). Electromyographic and skin temperature feedback provides information as to whether or not muscles are relaxing or skin temperature is increasing. There is considerable evidence that while the feedback is available, people can change the target response in the desired direction. Generalization of the skills is less easily produced.

In most cognitive-behavioral programs, cognitive strategies are added to basic relaxation skills. The range of particular techniques is wide. Three of the most common illustrate the approach. Self-instructional training teaches the patient coping statements that are rehearsed (19). For example, one man generated the following set of sentences: "What do I have to do when the pain starts to get worse? Well, I need to relax. I will resist taking a pill. If I distract myself, it won't seem so bad."

A second technique involves covert rehearsal and the imaginal activities (8). The individual practices desired responses, including coping with pain, by imagining the successful carrying out of the sequence. One woman who had not walked for several years covertly rehearsed walking up and down the hall unaided, pausing each time the pain went down her leg. In one of the last sessions, she walked down the hall unaided. Her explanation of her ability to do it credited the imaginary walks with overcoming her fear of falling. Several nerve blocks and a comprehensive exercise program were also perceived as crucial.

The third technique is perceptual restructuring or reinterpretation of the nociceptive stimuli (6,7). The patient develops an image of the area that is incompatible with pain, for example, that it is numb, or focuses on just one aspect of the stimulus, such as warmth. Many of the specific ideas are borrowed from work in hypnosis and pain. One patient who experienced the pain as hot, burning, and sharp in the middle of his lower back practiced concentrating just on the sensation of heat. He developed an image of the hot sharpness melting into a warm, relaxed heavy feeling in his whole lower back.

The behavioral reacting system also receives attention in a cognitive-behavioral program. Teaching the patient about learning and contingency management is another lecture. To give a piano concert at Carnegie Hall is not the first step in learning to play the piano. Many trials of practice are required to develop refined performance of new motor skills, and reinforcement is necessary. Overcoming avoidance behavior may be especially trying. Fordyce (12) has several useful suggestions for presenting learning phenomena to clients.

Arbitrary separation of thoughts, feelings, and behaviors is useful for analyzing and understanding the primary aim of a particular treatment technique. In practice, a treatment program is a smooth blend of techniques that have proved useful for the client. Furthermore, practice with new behaviors or exercise programs may depend on the pain relief provided by a nerve block in order that initial trials can be started.

The standard for inclusion of any technique in treatment is its efficacy. The ability to predict is too poor to allow decisions to be made without a clinical trial. Since the procedures are noninvasive and involve virtually no risk, an empirical approach can be adopted. Since this is contrary to the usual practice of medicine, an explanation to the patient is helpful. The patient's responsibility is to record and to practice. After a reasonable trial, a failed technique is discarded and another tried. The responsibility for developing a schedule to practice, identifying useful images, administering reinforcement, and so on, also rests with the patient.

Self-control and active participation are required and are counter to the usual passive modes of receiving injections, being operated on, or swallowing pills. Both types of intervention are potentially beneficial. In this sense, chronic pain treatment is similar to other chronic illness management; the patient must be an active and knowledgeable participant. Because of this, patients can be important resources for each other.

Do cognitive-behavioral methods work? Research is equivocal. Several factors contribute to this inconclusive state of affairs. A primary problem is the discrepancy between the sensible clinical use of the treatment and the requirements of a controlled experiment. In a careful research design, each patient must be treated the same, receiving comparable treatments in the same time span, with appropriate controls. The empirical clinical approach just described treats each patient with only those procedures that the client reports to be effective. Further, it is designed to be integrated with simultaneous use of other treatments. Turk and Genest (27) have recently reviewed the experimental literature and are encouraging in their conclusions regarding the role of cognitive-behavioral approaches in chronic pain.

REFERENCES

1. American Psychiatric Association (1968): *Diagnostic and Statistical Manual of Mental Disorders*, 2nd Ed. American Psychiatric Association, Washington, D.C.
2. American Psychiatric Association (1980): *Diagnostic and Statistical Manual of Mental Disorders (3rd Ed.) DSM III*, American Psychiatric Association, Washington, D.C.
3. Benson, H. B. (1975): *The Relaxation Response*. William Morrow & Co., Inc., New York.
4. Bonica, J. J. (1974): Organization and function of a pain clinic. In: *Advances in Neurology, Vol. 4*, edited by J. J. Bonica, pp. 433–443. Raven Press, New York.
5. Brena, S. F., Wolf, S. L., Chapman, S. L., and Hammonds, W. D. (1980): Chronic back pain: electromyographic, motion and behavioral assessments following sympathetic nerve blocks and placebos. *Pain*, 8:1–10.

6. Bresler, D. E. (1978): Self-control of pain: The use of relaxation and guided imagery in a self-help control program. In: *Pain Abstracts, Vol. 1*, p. 36. Second World Congress on Pain, IASP, Seattle, Washington.

7. Bresler, D. E. (1979): *Free Yourself from Pain*, Simon & Schuster, Inc. New York.

8. Cautela, J.R. (1977): The use of covert conditioning in modifying pain behavior. *J. Behav. Ther Exper. Psychiatr.*, 8:45–52.

9. Cummings, C., Evanski, P.M., Debenedetti, M. J., Anderson, E. E., and Waugh, T. R. (1979): Use of the MMPI to predict outcome of chronic pain. In: *Advances in Pain Research and Therapy, Vol. 3*, edited by John J. Bonica, J.C. Liebeskind, and D. G. Albe-Fessard, pp. 667–670. Raven Press, New York.

10. Dahlstrom, W. G., Welsh, G. S., and Dahlstrom, L. E. (1972): *An MMPI Handbook, Volume I: Clinical Interpretation*. University of Minnesota Press, Minneapolis.

11. DeGood, D. E. (1979): A behavioral pain-management program: expanding the psychologist's role in a medical setting. *Prof. Psychol.*, 10:491–502.

12. Fordyce, W. E. (1976): *Behavioral Methods for Chronic Pain and Illness*. C. V. Mosby Co., St. Louis, Missouri.

13. Fordyce, W. E. (1979): Environmental factors in the genesis of low back pain. In: *Advances in Pain Research and Therapy, Vol. 3*, edited by J.J. Bonica, J. C. Liebeskind, and D. G. Albe-Fessard, pp. 659–666. Raven Press, New York.

14. Greenhoot, J. H., and Sternbach, R. A. (1974): Conjoint treatment of chronic pain. In: *Advances in Neurology, Vol. 4*, edited by J. J. Bonica, pp. 595–603. Raven Press, New York.

15. Hilgard, E. K., and Hilgard, J. K. (1975): *Hypnosis in the Relief of Pain*. William Kaufmann, Inc., Los Altos, California.

16. Jacobson, E. (1938): *Progressive Relaxation*. University of Chicago Press, Chicago.

17. Kalla, J. M., and Brechner, T. F. (1978): The role of premorbid adjustment upon treatment outcome of chronic pain patients. In: *Pain Abstracts, Vol. 1*, p. 209. Second World Congress on Pain. IASP, Seattle, Washington.

18. Maruta, T., Swanson, D. W., and Swenson, W. M. (1979): Chronic pain: which patients may a pain-management program help? *Pain*, 7:321–329.

19. Meichenbaum, D. H. (1977): *Cognition and behavior modification: An integrative approach*. Plenum Press, New York.

20. Orne, M. T. (1974): Pain suppression by hypnosis and related phenomena. In: *Advances in Neurology, Vol. 4*, edited by J. J. Bonica, pp. 563–572. Raven Press, New York.

21. Peterson, L. E., and Gerson, P. D. (1975): *Changing Thoughts, Feelings, and Behaviors: A Common Sense Approach*, Worcester, Massachusetts.

22. Schultz, S.H., and Luthe, W. (1959): *Autogenic therapy*. Grune & Stratton, New York.

23. Shanfield, S. B., Heiman, E. M., Cope, N., and Jones, J. R. (1979): Pain and the marital relationship: psychiatric distress. *Pain*, 7:343–351.

24. Skinner, B.F. (1953): *Science and Human Behavior*. MacMillan Publishing Co. Inc. New York.

25. Sternbach, R. A. (1974): *Pain patients: Traits and treatments*. Academic Press, New York.

26. Swanson, D. W., Swenson, W. M., Maruta, T., and McPhee, M. C. (1976): Program for managing pain. 1. Program description and characteristics of patients. *Mayo Clin. Proc.*, 51:401–408.

27. Turk, D. C., and Genest, M. (1979): Regulation of pain: the application of cognitive and behavioral techniques for prevention and remediation. In: *Cognitive-Behavioral Interventions: Theory, Research, and Procedures*, edited by P. C. Kendall and S. D. Hollon, pp. 287–318. Academic Press, New York.

28. Waring, E. M., Weisz, G. M., and Bailey, S. I. (1976): Predictive factors in the treatment of low back pain by surgical intervention. In: *Advances in Pain Research and Therapy, Vol. 1*, edited by J. J. Bonica and D. Albe-Fessard. Raven Press, New York.

Chronic Low Back Pain, edited by
M. Stanton-Hicks and Robert Boas.
Raven Press, New York © 1982.

Concepts of Pain

John D. Loeser

*Department of Neurological Surgery, University of Washington,
Seattle, Washington 98195*

Physicians and patients usually harbor a concept of pain that involves a linkage between body damage and the pain reported by the patient. This is an inadequate concept that leads both physicians and their patients into unnecessary difficulties in the management of chronic pain. Tales of military exploits are replete with examples of soldiers who were unaware of their injury at the time it occurred but sought medical attention hours later when the fighting diminished. Beecher (1) pointed out a similar phenomenon among the wounded GIs at Anzio Beachhead in World War II: The request for narcotics was much less than was anticipated, because having a wound meant that one would be shipped out of the combat zone back to the U.S.A. The medical literature is now full of examples of patients who reported severe chronic pain and seemed to suffer from it, yet they were cured by such modalities as nonanalgesic drugs, psychotherapy, or resolution of litigation. The tissue–pathology based concept fails to explain why an animal or person with a damaged nervous system fails to respond to a harmful stimulus or how someone with no detectable tissue damage can report pain, as is seen in tic douloureux, the thalamic syndrome, or phantom limb pain.

We should discard such an inadequate approach to pain and utilize a more powerful model that will aid in the diagnosis and treatment of chronic pain patients. This model is based upon four concepts: *nociception*, *pain*, *suffering*, and *pain behavior*. These suffice to explain the known phenomena of acute and chronic pain and can help in our quest for a rational analysis of the human condition. The general concept of this model is that tissue damage leads to nociception, which usually leads to pain, which is one of the causes of suffering, which in turn may lead to pain behavior (Fig. 1). Physicians and patients' families respond to pain behavior, which is the only observable aspect of the pain process.

Nociception is defined as potentially tissue-damaging thermal or mechanical energy that impinges on the specialized nerve endings of A-delta and C fibers. Debates about the specificity of a pain-sensing system have abounded for 2,000 years, but now there is little question that all higher animals have a peripheral sensory system that is designed to convey to the central nervous system the existence of the hazard of tissue damage (2). Using differential blockade of large and small axons, it is possible to show that the detection of tissue damage is unaltered when

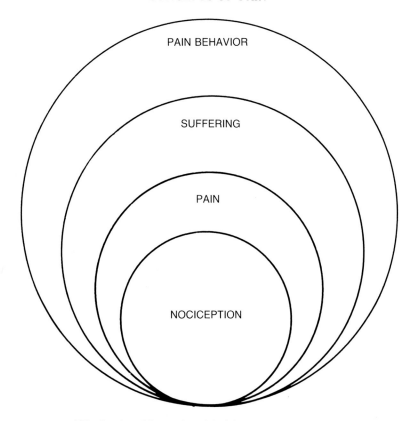

FIG. 1. A multifaceted model of the components of pain.

only the large axons are blocked, but that all response to tissue damage is abolished when the smaller A-delta and C fibers cannot conduct their impulses. Nociception is not an abnormal temporal or spatial activation of axons that normally transmit other types of information.

Nociception in the intact animal usually leads to *pain*, which I define as the perception of a nociceptive input to the nervous system. This is a circumscribed definition of pain and is not synonymous with any of the vernacular uses of the word. *Pain* has two important features: First, a nociceptive input must be perceived in order for it to become pain. If one is recording only from the A-delta and C fibers in the periphery, one cannot predict the organism's response without knowing a variety of other facts. Second, it is possible to perceive a nociceptive event even when no tissue-damaging energy has been imparted to the body. This is clinically obvious in such syndromes as tic douloureux, postherpetic neuralgia, postparaplegic pain, or the thalamic syndrome. These types of pain are reflections of alterations within the nervous system such that centrally conducting axons and their synapses are activated as if there had been a peripheral stimulus, when in fact no such stimulus has occurred. The clearest example of non-nociceptive pain is seen in in the absent part. Treatment strategies for pains caused by nervous system dysfunction ("central pains") must be different from those used to manage pain resulting from nociception. Surgical measures to eliminate nociceptive input further are not likely to relieve central pains, although they are often tried.

Suffering is a negative affective response generated in higher nervous centers by pain and other emotional situations, such as the loss of loved objects, stress, anxiety, or depression. It is essential to recognize that suffering is not uniquely related to pain, in spite of the fact that the language of pain is extensively utilized to refer to suffering. For example, an article in *Medical Economics* carried the title: "Can Quality Control Be This Painless?" A book entitled *Worlds of Pain: Life in the Working Class Family* was not concerned with peripheral nociceptors in the working people of America. We have all referred to someone as "a pain in the neck." Clearly we do not mean that the individual resides in our cervical region nor that there is nociceptive activity in that area. What we do mean is that someone else is causing us to suffer. Linguistic examples to support this concept are myriad.

Since suffering is a complex affective response, it is thoroughly integrated into an individual's life style. If we ignore the non-pain causes of suffering, we are likely to perpetuate the scenario described by Illich (3): "Medical civilization, however, tends to turn pain into a technical matter and thereby deprives suffering of its inherent personal meaning."

Suffering usually leads to *pain behavior*, which I define as any type of output from the organism that is commonly understood to suggest the existence of a tissue-damaging stimulus. Pain behaviors include but are not limited to talking, moaning, grimacing, limping, taking medicines, seeking health care, or refusing to work. In the absence of pain behaviors, we cannot ascertain that an individual is suffering. There is no reliable way of ascertaining the amount of someone's suffering, pain, or nociception; one can only quantify a variety of behaviors. All behaviors are, of course, generated by the brain, which is the organ of the mind. We can only infer the neural substrates of behavior.

It is essential to recognize that as we travel from nociception to pain to suffering to pain behavior, we must look outside of the individual organism; events that cannot be found within the patient play a significant role in the generation of pain behavior. It is obvious that loss of loved objects, depression, anxiety, or the effects of medication can lead to suffering and that the behavior manifested by the patient is indistinguishable from that caused by nociception. Finally, any behavior manifested over time is influenced by environmental responses. If one avoids an unpleasant job by low back pain, the symptoms may be impossible to ameliorate by therapies directed only at a presumed noxious stimulus.

All pain behavior is real; there is no such thing as "imagined" or "psychosomatic" pain. The Cartesian mind-body dualism is not a helpful concept when addressing patients with pain. The proper question is not "Does this patient hurt?" but "What are the factors which lead to this patient's pain behavior?" It is rare to find a patient with chronic pain that does not have multiple etiologic factors. Physicians tend to ignore the major roles of environmental factors in such patients. We blame much of our failure on one environmental factor—compensation—and ignore many others, such as the family, job satisfaction, life styles, and the amazingly deleterious effects of narcotics, sedative-hypnotics, and anti-anxiety drugs. We must expand our approaches to patients with chronic pain and replace the biomedical model with a learning-based model that includes all of the known contributors to chronic pain behavior. Specialists must learn to look beyond the technological aspects of their special interest areas and consider the patient as a whole person, subject not only to internal pathological processes but also to the stresses of his or her environment.

REFERENCES

1. Beecher, H. K. (1956): Relationship of significance of wound to pain experienced. *JAMA*, 161:1609–1613.
2. Collins, W. F., Neilsen, F. E., and Randt, C. T. (1960): Relation of peripheral nerve fiber size and sensation in man. *Arch. Neurol.*, 3:381–385.
3. Illich, I. (1976): *Medical Nemesis*. Random House, New York.

Chronic Low Back Pain, edited by
M. Stanton-Hicks and Robert Boas.
Raven Press, New York © 1982.

Strength Testing as a Method of Evaluating Ability to Perform Strenuous Work

W. Monroe Keyserling

*Department of Environmental Health Sciences Harvard School of Public Health,
Boston, Massachusetts 02115*

Reduction of the physical demands of particular jobs on the work force often calls for extensive engineering changes and may not always be feasible in existing plants. In these situations, an alternative and interim solution is to establish a program for selecting workers based on their ability to perform the strength requirements of their jobs.

This investigation was undertaken to develop a system for assessing workers' abilities to perform strenuous job elements. The specific objectives of this study were twofold: To use isometric strength tests to measure workers' strengths in simulation of strenuous job elements, and to determine the relationships among worker strength attributes, job requirements, and medical incidents.

METHODOLOGY

The investigation was a field study carried out in an aluminum smelting plant where a sample of employees assigned to entry level production jobs volunteered to participate. These jobs included the most physically demanding tasks found anywhere in the plant. The study was initiated in early 1977 and the data reported herein are current through summer 1979 (11). A longitudinal design was used to collect data. Major phases of the investigation are described below.

Biomechanical Job Analysis

The first step in collecting data was to evaluate biomechanically the strength requirements of the jobs under investigation. To do this, a 3-dimensional strength prediction model developed at the Ergonomics Laboratory of the University of Michigan was used. Complete details on this computerized model are available elsewhere. (1,6,10)

Job analyses were performed by a trained engineer from the participating plant. During the analysis, each job was systematically broken down into strenuous task elements. For each of these elements, the following variables were measured: (a) basic description of the task (e.g., lift, push, pull); (b) a description of the body posture maintained while performing the task (e.g., stand, sit, squat); (c) the force (in pounds) that was needed to perform the task; and (d) the location of the hands in space (with respect to the feet). These data were collected for both the starting and finishing positions and at points judged to be the most stressful during the trajectory of motion. Additional job analysis procedures have been described elsewhere.

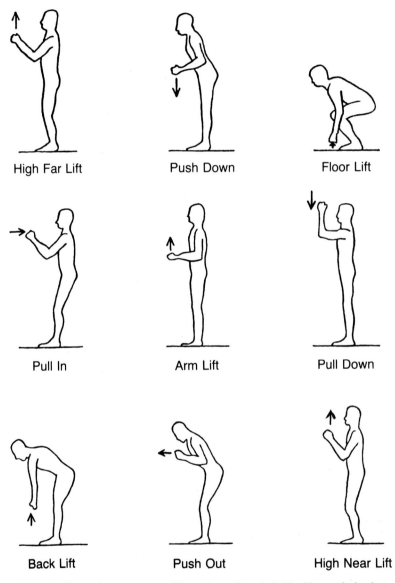

FIG. 1.   Strength test postures. (From Keyserling et al. (8) with permission.)

Design of Strength Tests

Following analysis of the entry-level jobs, the strength demands of several hundred tasks were documented. Of these, nine tasks were found to be of critical importance in terms of required strength (7). Strength tests were developed to simulate the postures and forces required to perform these tasks. These tests are illustrated in Fig. 1, and the corresponding jobs requirements are summarized in Table 1.

Strength Testing

Strength tests were administered to a cross-section of incumbent and new employees. Volunteers for the study were approved by the plant physician prior to taking the tests. All subjects performed a sustained (5 sec) maximum voluntary isometric exertion simulating each of the nine critical task elements shown in Table 1. The final 3 sec of the exertion were measured, and an average of this period was used to score performance. These procedures were consistent with *AIHA Ergonomics Guide* recommendations (2). In addition to strength measurements, employment and medical histories were recorded for each participant.

Medical Monitoring

At the time of strength testing, the medical record of each volunteer was tagged to indicate participation in the study. From this date forward, all visits to the medical department for job-related illness or injury were reported by the plant physician or the duty nurse.

RESULTS

A total of 344 workers (309 males, 35 females) participated in the study (8). Statistics (means, ranges, and standard deviations) computed on anthropomorphic

TABLE 1. *Description of critical strength elements*

| Test | Hand coordinates (cm) | | Critical element | Required force (Newtons) |
	Vertical	Horizontal		
High Far Lift	152	51	Lift pneumatic hammer	150
Push Down	112	38	Handle pot rake	400
Floor Lift	15	25	Lift lining	540
Pull In	157	33	Handle pot rake	310
Arm Lift	*	*	Lift TFR wheel	290
Pull Down	**	**	Handle hand jack	550
Back Lift	38	38	Lift steel hook	360
Push Out	124	36	Handle pot rake	270
High Near Lift	152	25	Lift huck gun	230

*Elbow at 90°, lower arm horizontal (See Fig. 1).
**Elbow at 90°, lower arm vertical (See Fig. 1).
Reprinted from Keyserling et al. (8) with permission.

measures (height, weight, and age) and strength scores for males and females are presented in Table 2.

During a monitoring period of approximately 26 months, 322 visits to the medical department were recorded. Table 3 presents a summary of incidents, days lost, and days restricted for each type of complaint.

To investigate the relationships among medical incidents, strength ability, and job demands, it was necessary to develop a simple quantitative relationship between strength-test performance and job-strength requirements. This was done by defining a new variable called the ability ratio (AR). It was calculated by dividing the force exerted on each strength test by the force required to perform the job:

$$AR = \frac{\text{Force on strength test}}{\text{Job requirement}}$$

TABLE 2. *Descriptive statistics—anthropometry and strength*

Measure	Males (n = 309)			Females (n = 35)		
	Mean	Range	SD	Mean	Range	SD
Height (cm)	180	152–201	6.6	168	152–180	6.9
Weight (kg)	83.5	57–132	12.4	71.9	54–100	10.7
Age	27.7	18–61	9.5	29.3	18–49	8.3
High Far Lift (N)	234	71–556	72	133	71–200	37
Push Down (N)	444	213–778	92	334	222–484	71
Floor Lift (N)	894	324–1689	243	552	191–1089	183
Pull In (N)	322	156–871	80	252	156–396	56
Arm Lift (N)	400	151–702	85	260	89–413	67
Pull Down (N)	608	382–925	101	452	253–649	105
Back Lift (N)	445	160–1360	154	316	178–636	113
Pust Out (N)	315	142–707	75	221	156–365	48
High Near Lift (N)	543	160–1138	156	282	133–596	100

N = Newton; n = number of subjects.
See Table 1 and Figure 1 for a description of test postures.
Reprinted from Keyserling et al. (8) with permission.

TABLE 3. *Summary of medical incidents*

Complaint type	Incident count	Days lost	Days restricted
Nonspecific	66	22	3
Skin contact	206	7	44
Musculoskeletal	50	7	18
Total	322	36	65

Reprinted from Keyserling et al. (8) with permission.

Ability ratios were computed on each of the nine strength tests for the 344 participants in the study. The job requirement (the denominator of the AR) was the force needed to perform the critical job element as simulated by the strength test (see Table 1).

Following the determination of ability ratios, employees were classified into the following three groups based on how well their strength abilities matched job demands: (a) weak, workers whose strength abilities were less than job-strength demands (AR < 0.75); (b), matched, workers whose strength abilities approximately equaled job demands (0.75 < AR < 1.25); and (c) strong, workers whose strength abilities exceeded job demands (AR > 1.25).

Although the above classification scheme was somewhat arbitrary, it was nonetheless consistent across all nine strength tests. In addition, it yielded adequate sample sizes for most of the analyses presented below.

Incidence rates, defined as the number of medical incidents per 200,000 hrs of job exposure (i.e., incidents/100 man-years) were determined for the weak, matched, and strong groups on each of the nine strength tests. These rates, which are presented in Table 4, were computed for all medical incidents and for those incidents classified as musculoskeletal.

To test for differences in the rates experienced by the groups, a Chi-square test was used (5,7). The results of the Chi-square analyses are also presented in Table 4. When the total number of medical visits was considered, employees who placed in the weak group for eight of the nine strength test categories suffered the highest incidence rates. The differences in rates were significant on four of the tests (the Pull In, Back Lift, Push Out, and High Near Lift). The weak group, determined by these tests, experienced between 1.25 and 2.71 times the incidence rates suffered by the matched and strong groups. Note that no consistent differences were found when the incidence rates experienced by the matched and strong groups were compared.

A similar analysis, presented on the right-hand side of Table 4, was performed on the 50 visits for musculoskeletal complaints. For these complaints employees who were in the weak group in six of the nine tests experienced the highest incidence rate, and the differences were significant for two (the Pull In and Back Lift). Employees in the weak group on these tests suffered between 1.6 and 3.1 times the musculoskeletal incidence rates of the other two groups. Test statistics could not be determined for either the Floor Lift or High Near Lift because the expected number of incidents (Exp) was insufficient.

DISCUSSION

In this study, a system was developed for identifying strenuous job elements and testing the strength of workers in simulations of these elements. Strength tests were administered to a cross-section of employees in an aluminum smelting plant, and they were also monitored for medical incidents.

As stated above, significant relationships were found among worker strength abilities, job demands, and medical incidents on four of the nine tests. Workers

TABLE 4. *Incidence rates by strength classification*

Test	Group	n	Exposure hours (× 1000)	All medical visits				Musculoskeletal visits			
				Obs.	Exp.	Rate	Test Stat. (Sig.)	Obs.	Exp.	Rate	Test Stat. (Sig.)
Hight Far Lift	Weak	16	71	21	15.2	59.2	2.42 (n.s.)	4	2.4	11.3	2.66 (n.s.)
	Matched	88	383	78	82.1	40.7		16	12.7	8.4	
	Strong	240	1049	223	224.7	42.5		30	34.9	5.7	
Push Down	Weak	21	93	29	19.9	62.4	4.53 (n.s.)	4	3.1	8.6	0.72 (n.s.)
	Matched	245	1071	220	229.4	41.1		33	35.6	6.2	
	Strong	78	339	73	72.6	43.1		13	11.3	7.7	
Floor Lift	Weak	12	53	15	11.4	56.6	1.18 (n.s.)	2	1.8	7.5	*
	Matched	78	343	73	73.5	42.5		15	11.4	8.7	
	Strong	254	1107	234	237.2	42.3		33	36.8	6.0	
Pull In	Weak	49	216	68	46.3	63.0	12.75 (.005)	13	7.2	12.0	6.35 (.05)
	Matched	236	1029	197	220.5	38.3		32	34.2	6.2	
	Strong	59	258	57	55.3	44.2		5	8.6	3.9	
Arm Lift	Weak	17	75	17	16.1	45.3	4.42 (n.s.)	3	2.5	8.0	3.88 (n.s.)
	Matched	115	508	126	108.8	49.6		23	16.9	9.1	
	Strong	212	920	179	197.1	38.9		24	30.6	5.2	
Pull Down	Weak	18	80	19	17.1	47.5	0.23 (n.s.)	6	2.7	15.0	4.52 (n.s.)
	Matched	260	1137	243	243.6	42.7		36	37.8	6.3	
	Strong	66	286	60	61.3	42.0		8	9.5	5.6	
Back Lift	Weak	31	136	44	29.1	64.7	19.43 (.001)	9	4.5	13.2	8.14 (.125)
	Matched	198	863	148	184.9	34.3		20	28.7	4.6	
	Strong	115	504	130	108.0	51.6		21	16.8	8.3	
Push Out	Weak	21	94	40	20.1	85.1	21.12 (.001)	5	3.1	10.6	1.26 (n.s.)
	Matched	210	914	179	195.8	39.2		30	30.4	6.6	
	Strong	113	495	103	106.0	41.6		15	16.5	6.7	
High Near Lift	Weak	6	27	15	5.8	111.1	16.46 (.001)	1	0.9	7.4	*
	Matched	26	116	30	24.9	51.7		9	3.9	15.6	
	Strong	312	1360	277	291.4	40.7		40	45.2	5.9	
Total		344	1503	322	—	42.8	—	50	—	6.65	—

*Expected value too small to compute x^2 statistic.
Reprinted from Magora (9) with permission.

whose strength abilities were less than job requirements suffered higher incidence rates than workers whose strength matched or exceeded job demands. Snook and his co-workers report that as many as two out of three overexertion injuries could be prevented by matching job-strength demands to population-strength abilities (12). The findings of this study indicate that similar reductions in medical incidents can be accomplished through a strength-testing program that matches the individual's strength ability to the strength demands of a job.

In addition to the significant correlations between strength and medical risk that were noted above, similar trends (i.e., weak workers suffering the highest incidence rates) were observed on four of the remaining five tests. The arm lift proved to be the exception. Here, matched workers experienced the highest incident rate. This finding should serve as a caution to those contemplating the use of strength tests for selecting workers. A pilot study should *always* be performed using incumbent employees; this will assure the validity of the tests before they are used for the selection of new employees.

The data reported herein reflect a relatively short monitoring period for medical incidents (only 26 months). Trauma on the musculoskeletal system from the performance of strength-demanding jobs may have cumulative effects that do not produce symptoms during early years of exposure. Only through long-term monitoring will these effects become apparent, and extended studies of this type are needed.

CONCLUSIONS

As stated at the beginning of this chapter, the desirable solution to the problem of handling materials manually is to redesign stressful jobs so that they will accomodate the physical capabilities of the work force. When this is done, selection procedures will not be needed, since it would be reasonable to assume that practically all applicants could safely and effectively perform all jobs. In the near future, however, this goal may not be technologically or economically feasible in all industries. Based on the findings of this and earlier studies (3,4), isometric strength testing is an effective and valid tool that can be used by industry as part of an employee selection and placement program.

REFERENCES

1. Chaffin, D. B. (1969): A computerized biomechanical model: Development of and use in studying gross body actions. *J. of Biomech.*, 2:429–441.
2. Chaffin, D. B. (1975): Ergonomics guide for the assessment of human strength. *Am. Ind. Hyg. Assoc. J.*, 36:505–510.
3. Chaffin, D. B. (1974): Human Strength Capability and Low Back Pain. *JOM*, 16(4):248–254.
4. Chaffin, D. B., Herrin, G. D., Keyserling, W. M., and Foulke, J. A. (1977): *Pre-Employment Strength Testing in Selecting Workers for Materials Handling Jobs.* NIOSH Physiology and Ergonomics Branch, Contract No. CDC-99-74-62, Cincinnati, Ohio.
5. Duncan, A. J. (1965): *Quality Control and Industrial Statistics.* Richard D. Irwin, Inc., Homewood, Illinois.
6. Garg, A., and Chaffin, D. B. (1974): A biomechanical computerized simulation of human strength. *AIIE Transactions*, 7(1):1–15.

7. Keyserling, W. M. (1979): *Isometric Strength Testing in Selecting Workers for Strenuous Jobs.* Ph.D. Dissertation, The University of Michigan, Ann Arbor, MI: University Microfilms International.

8. Keyserling, W. M., Herrin, G. D., Chaffin, D. B., Armstrong, T. J., and Foss, M. L. (1980): Establishing an Industrial Strength Testing Program. *Am. Ind. Hyg. Assoc. J.*, 41:730–736.

9. Magora, A. (1970): Investigation of the relation between low back pain and occupation. *Ind. Med. Surg.*, 39(12):28–34.

10. Schanne, F. J., Jr. (1972): *A Three-Dimensional Hand Force Capability Model for a Seated Person.* Ph.D. Thesis, The University of Michigan, Ann Arbor.

11. Snook, S. H. (1978): The Design of Manual Handling Tasks. *International Ergonomics Society Lecture—1978.* Bedfordshire, England.

12. Snook, S. H., Campanelli, R. A., and Hart, J. W. (1978): A study of three preventive approaches to low back injury. *JOM*, 20:478–481.

Chronic Low Back Pain, edited by
M. Stanton-Hicks and Robert Boas.
Raven Press, New York © 1982.

Anti-inflammatory Drug Therapy for Low Back Pain

Thomas G. Kantor

*Department of Medicine, New York University School of Medicine, New York,
New York 10016*

It is widely recognized that most back disorders treated by the average physician have no easily ascertainable etiology but are probably associated with greater or lesser degrees of inflammation. A similar situation exists with other rheumatological disorders and, therefore, the pharmacological weapons at the command of the rheumatologist are worthwhile considering as part of the armament available to the practitioner treating back disorders. Certain definitive rheumatological disorders can be fairly readily recognized, including ankylosing spondylitis, the back syndrome accompanying Reiter's syndrome, and those cases of juvenile rheumatoid arthritis with back inflammation that persist into adult life. These three entities may specifically be treated with indomethacin, phenylbutazone, and sulindac as the drugs of choice, although aspirin suffices for some patients.

It is, therefore, germane for us to review briefly what is known about inflammation and its control by pharmacological agents. A histological description of the inflammatory process may be summarized as follows:

Following an appropriate stimulus in the connective tissues, the surrounding capillary network first dilates and then becomes leaky with an exudation of plasma constituents out into the affected area. Leukocytes marginate against the inside wall of the endothelial lining of the capillaries and stick there. Soon thereafter, the leukocytes diapedese through openings between the endothelial cells out into connective tissue spaces, and more leukocytes are brought to the area by the circulation. The exact initiating and presumed humoral stimuli for the events up to this point are unknown, but they may be bacterially or virally induced materials, possibly kinins or prostaglandins. It is also possible that stimulation of local mast cells may produce histamine (7).

At any rate, once white cells are brought into the area, they begin to engulf the inflammation-inducing stimuli (such as bacteria or the already produced detritus of inflammation) into lysosomal packets and regurgitate some of the lysosomal enzymes out into the connective tissue milieu. These enzymes further amplify the inflammatory process where their lipidases produce prostaglandin end-products and their proteases produce kinins and complement products (35). From all these end-products, chemotactic signals are produced that bring more white cells into the area and continue the capillary dilatation and the leakage of plasma products, including antibodies and antibacterial materials, into the area.

The exact sequencing of signals, whether humoral or otherwise, that shuts down this process after it has been sufficiently advanced to succeed in eradicating the inflammatory stimulus or has failed to do so is still unknown. There is some evidence that both membrane stability and reactivity, as well as metabolic energy pathways, can be triggered by various inflammation mediators in such a way as to turn cell activity on and off (33). However, the exact sequence and control of such steps is still unknown.

Inflammation mediators that can accomplish all of the above histological steps are known to be a heterologous group, obviously so important to the organism that many back-up systems, some of them interconnected, are now known. These are described below.

MEDIATORS OF INFLAMMATION

The Kinin System

Kinins are nonapeptides that are produced by protease digestion of an alpha-globulin produced in the liver. Bradykinin is the best known (16).

The Prostaglandin System

After perturbation of bilayered membranes frees up the interior-pointing lipids, these compounds are digested by phospholipases to arachidonic acid. This, in turn, is acted upon by at least three enzyme systems, each with its own set of products (Fig. 1). The leukotrienes (HPETE and HETE) are intensely vasoactive materials that produce slow-reacting substance A, still another mediator of inflammation. Endoperoxides (PGG_2 and PGH_2), which survive only seconds or minutes, are known to be inflammation-mediating substances that are, in turn, acted upon by other enzymes to produce the more stable prostaglandin products. A third pathway produces chemotactic lipids and probably other active products of which we are still unaware (2).

The Complement Cascade

Total complement is a large molecular-weight plasma constituent that can be broken down by proteases into nine distinct components, some of which interact with each other to form complexes that perform all of the histologically important inflammation features noted above (26).

The Superoxide System

Throughout the prostaglandin synthesis pathway and in many other biological systems associated with inflammation, oxygenation by-products are produced, such as superoxide, singlet oxygen, and hydroxyl groups. All of these by-products are

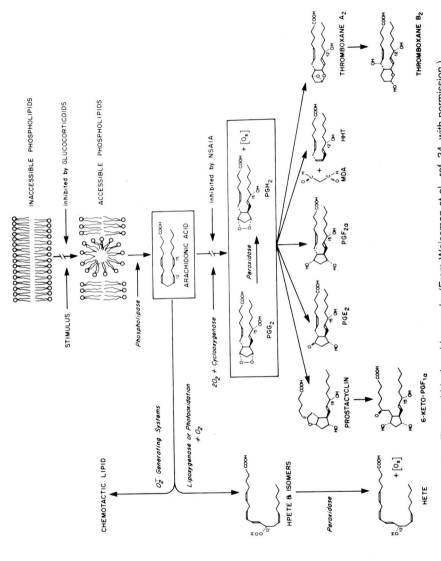

FIG. 1. The arachidonic acid cascade. (From Weissman et al., ref. 34, with permission.)

intensely toxic to membranes, and they are thought to be the materials primarily responsible for killing the bacterial cells that are ingested into leukocytes. However, these materials are also perfectly capable of killing living mammalian cells of their own species; we are protected from these products by the ubiquitous dismutases, which sponge up and neutralize these oxygen by-products almost as fast as they can be produced. Dismutases are usually high molecular-weight proteins that have copper and zinc ions associated with them (23). However, multivalent metallic cations in general may suffice.

Histamine, Serotonin, and Catecholamines

These are primarily vasoactive materials that can cause either dilatation or constriction of small arterioles and thereby control flow through the capillaries. They are produced from mast cells, platelets, and nerve endings in the inflammatory area, and the exact control of their activities in relation to inflammation is still unknown, although it is strongly suspected that they interact with the other mediators of inflammation (25).

ANTI-INFLAMMATORY DRUGS

All of the drugs to be discussed in this section interfere with cyclo-oxygenase, an enzyme involved in prostaglandin synthesis. Some of the drugs also have minor influences on the kinin system, and some indirectly affect the complement cascade by modifying immune mechanisms. Formation of immune complexes and activation of cellular immunity are common triggers of the complement cascade. As will be pointed out below, not one of these mechanisms adequately explains the anti-inflammatory effect of these drugs, which are all presumed to work in the peripheral site where the inflammation takes place. Quite probably related to this activity is the invariable analgetic effect of these drugs (15).

Salicylates

The oldest, best known, and least expensive of the anti-inflammatory drugs are the salicylates, aspirin in particular. The analgetic properties of salicylates were established over many centuries and culminated with the discovery of aspirin at the end of the 19th century. In the early part of this century, its anti-inflammatory capability was established.

Aspirin

Milligram for milligram, aspirin is the most potent of the salicylates, with respect both to its analgetic and its anti-inflammatory properties. A large number of metallic and organic salts of salicylic acid have also been developed; these require dosage levels far above that of aspirin to achieve an equivalent effect.

In dosages of less than 3.5 g/day, aspirin has primarily an analgetic effect with very little anti-inflammatory activity. However, at 3.5 g/day and more, a distinct anti-inflammatory effect can be demonstrated in a disease such as rheumatoid arthritis (1). Aspirin is extensively bound to serum albumin, but the degree of binding and therefore the concentration of the presumably pharmacologically active free portion seems to vary greatly from individual to individual. A total salicylate level (i.e., free and bound) of 15 mg % probably represents the onset of anti-inflammatory activity. At 30 mg%, tinnitus is almost always present in the adult, and at blood levels higher than 30 mg%, the central nervous system respiratory center is stimulated. This can lead to respiratory alkalosis and, at higher concentrations, to metabolic acidosis. Changes in mental affect almost invariably accompany these metabolic changes.

Aspirin has a direct toxic effect on the gastric mucosal cells, so that back diffusion of acid takes place, leading to cell death and to mucosal erosions (31). At anti-inflammatory dosage levels, such erosions almost invariably take place and lead to losses between 5 and 12 cc of blood daily. A healthy bone marrow can easily overcome such a loss. These erosions may be asymptomatic, but their presence is still the leading side effect of this drug, causing heart burn, nausea, and a feeling of abdominal fullness. To overcome this, various pharmaceutical strategies have been employed, such as buffering agents and enteric coating. These are more or less successful in reducing symptoms of gastric irritation, depending on the amount of buffer added or the effectiveness of the enteric coating (18).

In prescribing aspirin as therapy for inflammation, the physician must point out to the patient the analgetic and anti-inflammatory effects of the drug. The author has found it instructive to tell patients that the aspirin they take today will tend to prevent the inflammation they would have tomorrow. To assure this effect, it must be taken continuously in a set dose, irrespective of the patient's daily symptoms. At the end of 3 days of dosing, a steady state is achieved, after which salicylate blood levels taken at any time over the 24-hr period are generally similar (19).

It is useful for the clinician to understand that aspirin does not obey first-order kinetics in the sense that its elimination half-life is independent of the dose given. In actual fact, the elimination half-life of aspirin is dependent on the dose given and varies directly with the dose. A reason for this is that the main metabolic degradation product of aspirin is salicyluric acid, which depends on a conjugation of salicylate with glycine through an enzymatically controlled step. The enzyme responsible for this conversion has a finite capacity that becomes overloaded at a dosage of approximately 3.5 g/day (20). The addition of a few aspirin tablets beyond that point may increase the total salicylate serum concentration enough so that a patient tolerating 12 aspirin tablets daily but not achieving much of a therapeutic effect may do very much better with the addition of only one or two more tablets on a daily basis. Conversely, a patient taking 16 tablets daily with good therapeutic results but with a considerable degree of adverse effects may still do well if the dose is lowered by only one or two tablets; this reduction may bring the total dose within the capacity of the enzyme system that manufactures salicyluric acid.

Mechanism of action.

Aspirin is unique in its interference with the cyclo-oxygenase enzyme in that aspirin irrevocably changes the enzyme itself by the donation of an acetyl group. The enzyme must then be reconstituted in order that prostaglandin synthesis can continue (30). This is especially important with respect to the effect of aspirin on the platelet that, having separated from the megakaryocytes, no longer has a mitochondrial mechanism that can manufacture further protein products. Therefore, the effect of the drug on the platelet is irrevocable throughout the lifetime of the platelet, which is some 4 to 6 days.

Despite this powerful effect, it seems unlikely that aspirin's effect on inflammation can be entirely explained by the reduction of prostaglandin synthesis, since much higher doses are required to effect anti-inflammation than are required to turn off almost completely prostaglandin synthesis on a body-wide basis.

In addition to the direct toxic effect of aspirin on the stomach mucosa, there is another effect that adds to the potential for gastric irritation and ulcer formation. In addition to H_2 receptors as moderators of gastric physiology, prostaglandins also have a profound effect. Prostaglandins in the gastric mucosa reduce the production of acid and promote the mucosal blood supply and the production of the protective gastric mucus. Turning off prostaglandin production performs exactly the opposite effects, leading to more acid, less mucus, and a lower mucosal blood supply—a perfect situation for peptic ulcer production (28). All the other anti-inflammatory drugs to be discussed share this propensity, but only aspirin has a direct toxic effect on the mucosa.

The Phenylalkanoic Acids

The drugs in this category are all propionic acid derivatives; the first to be introduced was ibuprofen (Motrin) closely followed by fenoprofen (Nalfon) and naproxen (Naprosyn). All three interfere with prostaglandin synthesis by inhibiting cyclo-oxygenase but do so in a time-dependent fashion, so that upon withdrawal of the drug, the enzyme is often as good as new (29). Therefore, the pharmacokinetics of these drugs are of greater importance than that of aspirin, as far as this effect is concerned. These drugs also have some inhibitory effect on the kinin system and possibly the complement system as well (35). They do not seem to have antihistaminic effects. Their effect on the platelet is minimal when compared with aspirin.

The half-lives of ibuprofen and fenoprofen are between 1 and 3 hr, and they therefore require dosing on a t.i.d. or q.i.d. schedule at respective doses of 300 and 400 mg. More recent pharmacokinetic studies suggest the possibility of a two-compartment model that might allow b.i.d. dosing with higher than conventional single doses (5). Whether such schedules will change the adverse effect profiles or maintain effectiveness has yet to be demonstrated. Ibuprofen has been successfully prescribed by some rheumatologists at daily doses of 4200 mg.

All of these drugs have similar adverse effects in regard to gastric irritation as noted above, and they share with aspirin the potential for causing dependent edema by interfering with salt and water excretion by the kidney and enhancing the effect of antidiuretic hormone. These latter two effects are also under prostaglandin control (22). Secondary to the salt and water effects is a change in the water content of the cornea and lens of the eye with resultant effects on vision. More profound effects on the kidney have been reported, but rarely (4), and the incidence of drug-induced rashes is also low.

Naproxen, which shares the above side effects, has a half-life between 11 and 13 hr and therefore may be given on a 250 mg b.i.d. or once-a-day schedule. There seems to be little to choose among the three drugs except that the established b.i.d. dosage schedule for naproxen leads to better compliance on a long-term basis and may account for its preference by some investigators (14).

A disturbing theme that runs through all discussions of these drugs is the fact that the lack of effect of one drug in one chemical class in an individual patient does not necessarily imply that another one will not work. In addition, whereas a therapeutic effect from aspirin may well be noted within a 3-day period, the propionic acid derivatives may require a minimum of 10 days and possibly 3 weeks before a full therapeutic effect can be distinguished. It may therefore be necessary to take the better part of 2 months to determine which propionic acid derivative is most effective and least toxic for an individual patient.

Pyroles

The most familiar representative of this group of drugs is indomethacin. The pyroles are characterized by a five-membered ring containing a nitrogen. This configuration gives these drugs some resemblance to serotonin, which may account for some of the adverse effects noted with these drugs. A related compound, tolmetin (Tolectin), is also available, and another, zomepirac (Zomax), is being marketed as an oral analgesic. All members of this group are potent inhibitors of prostaglandin synthesis by their inhibition of cyclo-oxygenase, and they also have some modifying effects on the kinin system. Indomethacin's potent inhibition of prostaglandin synthesis has been utilized in areas other than that of anti-inflammation. It is a fairly potent, quick-acting analgetic agent (32). It controls the renal defect in Bartter's syndrome, which results from overactivity of the prostaglandins in the renal tubule (12). In the newborn, the drug can close a patent ductus arteriosus whose patency is maintained by prostaglandins that are inappropriately still being manufactured in the vessel after birth (13). In some instances, indomethacin can interfere with the leaching of bony matrix outside the periphery of bone metastasis, particularly in renal cell carcinoma, thereby reducing pain and hypocalcemia (3).

As an anti-inflammatory drug, indomethacin may be used in dosages of 75 to 200 mg/day given in divided doses t.i.d. or q.i.d. In addition to the gastric and renal problems, which it shares with all other anti-inflammatory drugs as adverse effects, indomethacin may also cause a peculiar vascular type of headache, particularly after the first morning dose, and may cause psychotomimetic effects. These latter two adverse effects may be related to the drug's serotonin-like configuration. Indomethacin has an elimination half-life of approximately 3 hr, and any single dose is excreted from the body within 12 hr.

Although milligram for milligram, tolmetin is probably slightly less potent than indomethacin, it is still a very effective anti-inflammatory drug in doses of 800 to 1200 mg. Its elimination half-life has been found to fit a two-compartment model with an initial phase of 1 hr and a second phase of 4 to 6 hr. This suggests that the drug is more lipid-soluble than indomethacin. However, to maintain peak plasma effects at least a t.i.d. dosage is probably indicated, although if high single doses are tolerated, it may be possible to give the drug b.i.d. (11). In anti-inflammatory dosage, the drug definitely has fewer side effects than indomethacin and is recommended for use in children, in contradistinction to indomethacin, which may be hepatotoxic in children.

Zomepirac, also a pyrole, is available as a potent oral analgetic agent. In single-dose analgetic trials, its potency approaches that of injected narcotics or oral Percodan (P. Stewart, McNeil Laboratories, *personal communication*).

Pyrazoles

The most characteristic pyrazole is phenylbutazone (Butazolodine), a very potent anti-inflammatory drug with severe adverse effects that are mostly dose dependent. Attempts to improve on phenylbutazone by chemical configurational changes that maintain its potency and eliminate its adverse effects have been unrewarding. A metabolite, oxyphenbutazone (Tandearil), has been disappointing (with respect to the reduction of adverse effects.) Both drugs inhibit prostaglandin synthesis, and phenylbutazone seems to have the added effect of specifically inhibiting the further metabolism of the endoperoxide most responsible for free-radical production (17). The effect on other inflammation-mediating pathways is uncertain, but the potency of the anti-inflammatory effect of these two drugs is certainly well beyond their effect on prostaglandin synthesis.

In addition to the usual adverse effects seen with the anti-inflammatory drugs, phenylbutazone is the most potent salt-retaining compound of the group to the extent that it should be given only with caution to patients with high blood pressure and borderline congestive heart failure (9). Ordinary diuretics seem to reverse most of the prostaglandin-induced effect on the kidneys. Also, both phenylbutazone and oxyphenbutazone may be toxic to bone marrow to an extent that is mostly dose dependent. However, there have been a few reports of idiosyncratic bone marrow wipe-outs from one or two doses of these drugs, however, this is very rare. Psychotomimetic effects may also be induced, perhaps related to the fact that pyrazoles contain five-membered rings with two nitrogens.

As noted above, indomethacin and phenylbutazone may almost seem specific for inflammatory spondyloarthropathies. Often, dosages of phenylbutazone no greater than 200 mg/day suffice to put a patient with ankylosing spondylitis at ease (27). Many patients tolerate 400 mg/day for prolonged periods, but such a dosage should be carefully monitored by examination of the blood and urine and blood pressure at fairly frequent intervals. A week-long trial of phenylbutazone with a 600 mg loading dose daily for 2 days and then 400 mg doses daily for 5 more days will often suffice to rule in or out the efficacy of this drug in an individual patient, with very little toxicity to concern the physician in that period of time.

Thiazines

Thiazines are interesting chemical entities as drugs. Some of them are hypo-glycemic agents and others are major tranquilizers, but there is also a group with anti-inflammatory effects. An original member of this group, fenclozic acid, was introduced into the British market for a short period of time but proved to be very toxic to the liver. Various modifications of the thiazine formula resulted in the drug sudoxicam, which had fairly potent anti-inflammatory effects but also was hepa-totoxic. The search for drugs in this category has culminated in the finding of piroxicam, an inhibitor of prostaglandin synthesis and an anti-inflammatory drug of moderate potency. Piroxicam has the interesting property of having a very [*FELDENE* handwritten] prolonged half-life, so that a single dose will suffice on a daily basis (E. M. Wiseman, Pfizer Laboratories, *personal communication*). This drug will soon be introduced into the American market. At a dosage of 20 mg daily, a good anti-inflammatory effect has been demonstrated in populations of rheumatoid patients. At lower dosages, this effect is very much reduced. The usual adverse effects for all prostaglandin-synthesis inhibitors are apparent with piroxicam to about the same extent as other drugs in this general category. However, dosages of piroxicam higher than 20 mg/day seem to be associated with an inordinately high incidence of proven peptic ulcer. One, therefore, seems to be locked in to the 20 mg daily dose; this at least satisfies the problem of compliance, which should be easy with this drug.

Sulindac

The drug sulindac (Clinoril) was introduced into the American market in late 1979 and proved an instant success because of a well-developed public relations campaign. The drug is unusual in that it is not active but must be reduced to a sulfide in the body before becoming effective. It is this metabolite, with a half-life of 13 hr, that is the active form of the drug. Another metabolite, a sulfone, is inactive but readily enters into the enterohepatic circulation and may cause diarrhea in certain patients, sometimes to a degree that necessitates discontinuing the drug (6). Sulindac is slightly related to the pyroles and also reduces prostaglandin syn-thesis; thus, it has the usual adverse effects associated with this action. The dosage schedule of 150 to 200 mg b.i.d. seems satisfactory for many people, and the incidence of adverse effects is no better or worse than other prescription anti-inflammatory drugs. The drug is also recommended for ankylosing spondylitis.

Fenamates

Mefenamic acid (Ponstel), from this chemical group, was introduced into the United States some years ago and proved to bring about certain renal changes that caused the Food and Drug Administration to limit its use to no more than 7 days duration. Since anti-inflammatory agents are sometimes meant to be utilized over periods of months and years, this restriction greatly limited the drug's use. It, too, interferes with prostaglandin synthesis at the site of the cyclo-oxygenase enzyme.

Meclofenamate (Meclamin), a very recently approved member of this chemical group, has anti-inflammatory features similar to the drugs noted above with a possibly slightly higher incidence of gastrointestinal side effects. At least it is a different chemical entity from any of the other anti-inflammatory drugs, which may form its main advantage.

Genetics of Anti-inflammatory Therapy

One very puzzling aspect of the use of these drugs is the inability of the physician to predict which patient will respond best to what drug. Thus, even drugs within the same chemical class, such as the propionic acids or the pyroles, may affect individual patients quite differently with respect to both the effectiveness and the promotion of adverse effects. If anti-inflammatory drug therapy is decided upon, the physician may have to run through several months of trial and error in order to find an optimum drug for an individual patient.

There are several possible explanations of this phenomenon. First, the study of pharmacogenetics demonstrates that there may be differences in the way individual patients absorb and metabolize drugs. No such differences have as yet been demonstrated among the anti-inflammatory drugs, although it has been noted that an esterase, which removes the acetyl group from aspirin, is in much higher concentrates in males than in females (24). It has been shown empirically that females, irrespective of their body surface area or weight, seem to get a greater pharmacological effect from aspirin than do males. Second, it is possible that there are genetic differences in the ways that individual subjects mount an inflammatory process, some perhaps using one mediating pathway more than another. Our understanding of such a phenomenon is in its infancy. Third, it is possible that at various stages of a disease process associated with inflammation, certain inflammatory pathways may be used preferentially over others. We have no information on this point nor do we know enough about which mediating pathways are most affected by the drugs in this category, with the possible exception of the effect on prostaglandin synthesis.

Until such questions as the above can be answered—and attempts are now being made—it will not be possible to predict with any accuracy how an individual patient will respond to any drug in this group. Therefore, it is probably wisest to begin with aspirin before prescribing any of the other more expensive drugs.

Mode of Action of Anti-inflammatory Drugs

The exact mode of action of the anti-inflammatory drugs discussed above is essentially unknown. We know that they work in the periphery to produce their analgetic effects (21) and, it is presumed, their anti-inflammatory effect as well. All of the drugs discussed above interfere with prostaglandin synthesis but it is unlikely that this is their sole mode of action (10). Entities such as EDTA, alpha-tocopherol, and chlorpromazine are all inhibitors of prostaglandin synthesis and are not considered to be potent anti-inflammatory agents. In addition, as has been noted, much smaller doses of these drugs inhibit prostaglandin synthesis universally whereas much higher doses are necessary to demonstrate a clinical anti-inflammatory effect.

A second possibility is the fact that almost all the drugs in this category uncouple oxidative phosphorylation at the mitochondrial site (8). However, this effect cannot be demonstrated in whole cells, and the most potent uncoupler of oxidative phosphorylation known is thyroxine, which is not held to have anti-inflammatory effects. If it was an important feature in the action of these drugs, this enzymatic step would produce energy that would be necessary for the mounting of an inflammatory response and thus interference with it would seriously impede the production of inflammation.

A third theory is that, just as there is an endogenous morphine-like substance, there may be an endogenous anti-inflammatory substance, possibly augmented by anti-inflammatory drugs, in apposition to the inflammation-producing mediators. Such a phenomenon would not be inconsistent with our knowledge of the positive and negative controls of many biological mechanisms. However, a wide search for such a substance has been unrevealing, although PGE_1, a prostaglandin end-stage product, has been shown to have anti-inflammatory properties (7). However, the demonstration of this requires enormous doses unlikely to be found even in local areas of the body.

A fourth possibility is that the drugs interfere with leucocyte function and/or mobility. The problem here is that, depending on the models utilized by different investigators, different results are found, and even in the same laboratory, results may not be reproducible. Until a good model system has been devised to test drugs with respect to their ability to inhibit leucocyte activities, such as pinocytosis, cell-membrane receptor activity, or mobility, it will be difficult to characterize drugs with these properties or to devise specifically new drugs.

It is perhaps best to admit simply that we don't know how these drugs work, and until our understanding of the inflammation process increases and our ability to test drugs within the framework of a full understanding of inflammation becomes available, we shall be sorely handicapped in our ability to prescribe drugs for anti-inflammatory effect.

In summary, anti-inflammatory drugs can and should be used in the treatment of back complaints if only for their universal analgetic effect. Trial and error will determine the drug and dosage to be used. Tolerance does not occur with prolonged use, and certain inflammatory back conditions can be treated specifically with these drugs.

REFERENCES

1. Bayles, T. B. (1972): Salicylate therapy for rheumatoid arthritis. In: *Arthritis and Allied Conditions*, edited by J. L. Hollander and D. J. McCarty, Jr., ch. 28. Lea & Febriger, Philadelphia, Pennsylvania.
2. Bergstrom, S. (1967): Prostaglandins: Members of a new hormonal system. *Science*, 157:382–391.
3. Brereton, H. D., Halushka, P. V., Alexander, R. W., Mason, D. M., Keiser, H. R., and DeVito, V. T., Jr. (1974): Indomethacin responsive hypocalcemia in a patient with renal cell adenocarcinoma. *N. Engl. J. Med.*, 291:83–85.
4. Brezin, J. H., Katz, S. M., Schwartz, A. B., and Chinitz, J. L. (1979): Reversible renal failure and nephrotic syndrome associated with non-steroidal anti-inflammatory drug. *N. Engl. J. Med.*, 301:1271–1273.
5. Brugueras, N. E., LeZotte, L. A., and Moxley, T. E. (1978): Ibuprofen: A double-blind comparison of twice-a-day therapy with four-times-a-day therapy. *Clin. Therap.*, 2:13–21.
6. Duggan, D. E., Hare, L. E., Ditzier, C. A., Lei, B. W., and Kwan, K. C. (1977): The disposition of sulindac. *Clin. Pharm. Therap.*, 21:326–335.
7. Ebert, R. H. (1965): The experimental approach to inflammation. In: *The Inflammatory Process*, edited by B. W. Zweifach, L. Grant and R. T. McCluskey, ch. 1. Academic Press, New York.
8. Famaey, J. P. (1975): More recent non-steroidal anti-inflammatory drugs. Part 1: Mode of action. *Clin. Rheum. Dis.*, 1:285–306.
9. Famaey, J. P., Brooks, P. M., and Dick, W. C. (1975): Biologic effects of non-steroidal anti-inflammatory drugs. Seminars. *Arthritis Rheum.*, 5:63–81.
10. Glenn, E. M., Bowman, B. J., and Rohloff, N. A. (1979): Anomalous biological effects of salicylates and prostaglandins. *Agents Actions*, 9:257–264.
11. Grindel, J. M., Migdalof, B. H., and Plostnieks, J. (1979): Absorption and excretion of tolmetin in arthritic patients. *Clin. Pharmacol. Therap.*, 26:122–128.
12. Halushka, P. V., Wohltmann, H., Privitera, P. J., Hurwitz, G., and Margolius, H. S. (1977): Bartter's Syndrome: Urinary prostaglandin E-like material and kallikrein; Indomethacin effects. *Ann. Int. Med.*, 87:281–286.
13. Heymann, M. A., Rudolph, A. M., and Silverman, N. H. (1976): Closure of the ductus arteriosus in premature infants by inhibition of prostaglandin synthesis. *N. Engl. J. Med.*, 295:530–533.
14. Huskisson, E. C., Woolf, D. L., Balme, H. W., Scott, J., and Franklyn, S. (1976): Four new anti-inflammatory drugs: Responses and variations. *Brit. Med. J.*, 1:1048–1049.
15. Kantor, T. G. (1979): Ibuprofen. *Ann. Int. Med.*, 91:877–882.
16. Kantor, T. G., Jarvik, M. E., and Wolff, B. B. (1967): Bradykinin as a mediator of human pain. *Proc. Soc. Exper. Biol. Med.*, 126:505–506.
17. Kuehl, F. A., Jr., Humes, T. L., Egan, R. W., Ham, E. A., Beveridge, G. C., and Van Arman, C. G. (1977): Role of prostaglandin endoperoxide PGG_2 in inflammatory processes. *Nature (New Biol.)*, 265:170–175.
18. Lanza, F. L., Royer, G. L., and Nelson, R. S. (1980): Endoscopic evaluation of the effects of aspirin, buffered aspirin and enteric coated aspirin on gastric and duodenal mucosa. *N. Engl. J. Med.*, 303:136–138.
19. Levy, G. (1979): Pharmacokinetics of salicylate in man. *Drug. Metab. Rev.*, 9:3–19.
20. Levy, G., Amsel, L. P., and Elliott, H. E. (1969): Kinetics of salicyluric acid elimination in man. *J. Pharm. Sci.*, 58:827–829.
21. Lim, R. K. S. (1968): Neuropharmacology of pain and analgesia. In: *Pharmacology of Pain*, Vol. 9, edited by R. K. S. Lim, D. Armstrong and E. G. Pardo. Pergamon Press, Oxford.
22. Lum, G. M., Aisenbrey, G. A., Dunn, M. J., Berl, T., Schrier, R. W., and McDonald, K. M. (1977): In vivo effect of indomethacin to potentiate the renal medullary cyclic AMP response to vasopression. *J. Clin. Invest.*, 59:8–13.
23. McCord, J. M., and Fridovich, I. (1978): The biology and pathology of oxygen radicals. *Ann. Int. Med.*, 89:122–127.
24. Menguy, R., Desbaillets, L., Masters, Y. F., and Okabe, S. (1972): Evidence for a sex linked difference in aspirin metabolism. *Nature (New Biol.)*, 239:102–103.

25. Morrell, R. M. (1970): Neuroendocrine mechanisms in inflammation. *Excerpta Medica International Congress Series*, 229:269–283.
26. Muller-Eberhard, H. J. (1978): Complement abnormalities in human disease. *Hosp. Pract.*, 13:65–76.
27. Ogryzlo, M. (1972): Ankylosing Spondylitis. In: *Arthritis*, 8th ed., edited by J. L. Hollander and D. J. McCarty, Jr., ch. 41. Lea & Febriger, Philadelphia, Pennsylvania.
28. Robert, A. (1974): Effects of prostaglandins on the stomach and the intestine. *Progstaglandins*, 6:523–532.
29. Rome, L. H., and Lands, W. E. M. (1975): Structural requirements for time dependent inhibition of prostaglandin biosynthesis by anti-inflammatory drugs. *Proc. Natl. Acad. Sci.*, 72:4863–4865.
30. Roth, G. J., Stanford, N., and Majerus, P. W. (1975): Acetylation of prostaglandin synthase by aspirin. *Proc. Natl. Acad. Sci.*, 72:3073–3076.
31. Smith, B. M., Skillman, J. J., Edwards, B. G., and Silen, W. (1971): Permeability of the human gastric mucosa. Alteration by acetylsalicylic acid and ethanol. *N. Engl. J. Med.*, 285:716–721.
32. Sunshine, A., Laska, E., Meisner, M., and Morgan, S. (1964): Analgesic studies of indomethacin as analyzed by computer techniques. *Clin. Pharm. Therap.*, 5:699–707.
33. Weissmann, G., Dukor, P., and Zurier, R. B. (1971): Effect of cyclic AMP on release of lysosomal enzymes from phagocytes. *Nature (New Biol.)*, 231:131–135.
34. Weissmann, G., Korchak, H. M., Perez, H. D., Smoler, J. E., Goldstein, I. M., and Hoffstein, S. T. (1979): Leukocytes as secretory organs of inflammation. In: *Advances in Inflammation Research, Vol. 1*, edited by G. Weissman, R. Paoletti, and B. Samuelsson, pp. 111. Raven Press, New York.
35. Weissmann, G., Smolen, J. E., and Korchak, H. M. (1980): Release of inflammatory mediators from stimulated neutrophils. *N. Engl. J. Med.*, 303:27–34.
36. Willkens, R. F. (1974): The mechanisms of action of anti-inflammatory agents in the control of pain. In: *Advances in Neurology*, edited by J. J. Bonica, pp. 547–555. Raven Press, New York.
37. Zurier, R. B., and Quagliata, F. (1971): Effect of prostaglandin E on adjuvant arthritis. *Nature (New Biol.)*, 234:304–305.

Chronic Low Back Pain, edited by
M. Stanton-Hicks and Robert Boas.
Raven Press, New York © 1982.

Physical Modalities and Low Back Pain Management

Rene Cailliet

Department of Rehabilitative Medicine, University of Southern California School of Medicine, Los Angeles, California 90033

In most episodes of acute low back pain, recovery is spontaneous. However, during the acute phase, there are numerous modalities that decrease or may even eliminate the pain. Various of these physical therapies are used in an attempt to shorten the acute episodes, maintain function, prevent secondary factors that contribute to pain and disability, and decrease the progression to chronic low back pain. Sometimes pain that persists in spite of intensive treatment with physical modalities, medication, modification of activities, and injection techniques may develop into a syndrome of chronic pain. Once established, the occurrence of pain or its intensification may no longer be related to nociceptive peripheral stimuli emanating from tissues considered to be the pain source. At this phase, a movement or position that is expected to cause or aggravate pain is no longer necessary, and the traditional somatic treatments may no longer be of value, leading to controversy concerning the anatomy and pathophysiology of the chronic low back pain disorder (6).

ROLE OF PHYSICAL THERAPIES

In the acute, usually limited episodes of low back pain, the techniques offer relief or diminution of pain while the patient makes a spontaneous recovery. General anxiety, impaired function, and immobility are more rapidly curtailed ensuring faster and probably more complete recovery.

In recurrent low back pain, a mechanical factor is usually present; once that is identified, the patient needs assistance and training to avoid aggravating movement or exercises to facilitate the accomplishment of the proper movement. Modalities may be used to facilitate exercise to ensure this end result.

For chronic low back pain, various modalities are used to decrease either the perception of pain or decrease the intensity of nociceptive impulses that may reinitiate or intensify various pain cycles. Although many of these modalities have limited value in this respect in that they are not necessarily curative nor fully effective nor understood in their mode of action, they nevertheless have proven value and are accepted by both patient and physician in aiding low back pain management.

In many instances, several physical modalities may be used concurrently and in conjunction with other forms of definitive therapy.

Before undertaking any form of physical management, as with any other therapy, a thorough evaluation of the patient and his physical and subjective presentation must be assessed to determine the most appropriate therapy.

PATIENT EVALUATION

In evaluating any patient with back pain, the tissue site of pain origin is sought within the function unit of the lumbar or lumbosacral spine region. This tissue site is determined by inspection, palpation, and specific segmental movement of the spine—both active and passive—at each functional unit, which is one of six segments of the lumbosacral spine. The functional unit here is defined as two adjacent vertebrae with their interposed intervertebral disk and with all the contiguous tissues such as ligaments, bones, articulations with their synovium, cartilage, capsules, muscles, blood vessels, and all related nerves (3).

The tissues that have been confirmed to be sensitive to noxious stimulation are the anterior longitudinal ligaments, the posterior longitudinal ligament, the outer annular fibers of the intervertebral disks, the nerves with their dural sheath, the posterior erector spinae muscles, the facet joint capsules, the interspinous ligaments, the skin, and the bony periosteum. Confirmation of which of these tissues that are being irritated and of the mechanism by which this has occurred constitutes the basis of a meaningful examination and correct treatment choice (4).

Successful treatment demands either that the cause of irritation be removed or reduced or that the nervous system response be modified. Failure to accomplish one of these goals in the early phase may result in prolonged disability, development of secondary complications, or recurrence of acute pain, which gradually progresses into a chronic syndrome.

PHYSICAL THERAPY MODALITIES AND THEIR USE

Sensory Stimulation Techniques

Somatosensory inputs labeled as counterirritants or hyperstimulation algesia have been effective in reducing pain. Both clinical and experimental evidence demonstrates that heat, cold, stroking, intense pressure, electrical stimulation, and acupuncture can decrease pain. Various hypotheses based on gate modulation and neurotransmitter release have been proposed as the mediators of this response.

Cryotherapy

Applications of ice or cold have been extensively used and have proved to be a valuable adjunct for treating low back pain (7,11). Cryotherapy works best in relieving superficial rather than deep pain, particularly in acute disorders, but recently it has been advocated by Melzack et al. (12) as being effective in relieving chronic back pain also.

Cold utilization for low back pain therapy is provided by applying ice or a cold spray to the skin centrally or over the paraspinal muscles (2,9,13). A broad sweeping motion is advocated with ethyl chloride or a vasocoolant spray applied to the skin along the direction of the underlying muscle. A similar motion across the skin with ice cubes is also considered the ideal way to use this modality. Immediately after completing these applications, the muscle should be stretched gently, both passively and actively.

Several short treatment sessions are best because continuous application of cold to a muscle can gradually cause ischemia which, in turn, results in greater irritability and thus greater pain. Use of cold applications to provide analgesia may work by means of a segmental gating mechanism or possibly by means of cold activating brain stem mechanisms that are now considered to exert descending inhibitory influences on pain signals; this activation is similar to that caused by electrical stimulation or acupuncture activation of ventricular gray areas (5). Ice also probably acts upon the spindle system of the muscles that are considered to be in spasm as protection against movement of the painful functional unit (1). This spasm may also occur as a primary reaction to direct trauma or as a response to acute articular inflammation of the facet joint, irritation of the posterior primary division, or vasomotor changes. Although muscle spasm is essentially a protective immobilization of the irritated inflamed functional unit, the spasm itself may ultimately become the nidus of pain from prolonged muscular contraction.

When microscopic hemorrhage from trauma occurs within the muscle, application of ice may abort further hemorrhaging. Frank hemorrhage is rare in the usual presentation of mechanically induced low back pain, but microscopic hemorrhage or edema is probably more frequent than is suspected.

Heat

Applied locally to skin and back muscle, heat is also considered to be beneficial in that it too decreases muscle spasm and modifies the nociceptive afferent impulse. Heat allegedly increases the blood supply to the muscle, facilitating oxygenation of the tissues and elimination of metabolic products that have been created by sustained muscle contraction.

Heat can be applied in various forms, such as hot moist compresses, exposure to large electric light bulbs, diathermy, microthermy, and infrared and short-wave diathermy. Ultrasound is also advocated as a form of deep heat, especially when increased circulation of deeper tissues is sought. Moist heat is considered to be the most effective and is widely employed in the form of direct applications or heat baths, providing good heat transfer with convection and conduction through the tissues.

As with the use of various cold therapies, heat is best employed with other modalities of therapy, especially prior to exercising in order to overcome ischemia and muscle contraction, thus allowing better muscle function and range of movement during therapy.

Massage

Depending on the type of massage, a specific effect can be elicited by creating sensory stimulation, increasing blood flow, stretching tissues, or causing counter-irritation. When massage is used for sensory stimulation, it has the same efficacy and indications as the application of heat, ice, or electrical stimulation. Massage of the kneading type enhances vasomotor and lymphatic drainage.

Manipulation

Manipulation or mobilization is a manually applied mechanical stretch of a specific tissue site. Essentially, manipulation is directed at influencing the relationship and the integrity of an articulation. In spinal manipulation, the force effect is primarily upon the posterior zygoapophyseal joints with effect also on the intervertebral joint and all the contiguous tissue (10).

The effects of joint manipulation remain controversial. The ultimate goal beyond relief of pain is to return lost motion of the joint to permit segmental movement. Mennell (10) has claimed that the technique does result in regaining "joint play" and indicates that restoring function around and beyond the joint range can be achieved by both active and passive movements. This added range of motion is considered to be physiological and necessary for normal pain-free point movement. Loss of joint motion is considered to result from faulty movement, trauma, imbalance, protective muscular spasm, emotional tension, or degenerative articular changes. All of these and more play a part.

Joint dysfunction, causing local inflammation or mechanical encroachment to contiguous tissues, may irritate the nerve root in that vicinity. Pain in the distribution of the posterior primary division may result, and sympathetic vasomotor changes may result as well (8). Regaining motion of that joint may remove or reduce the irritation encroaching on the nerve roots.

Other explanations for the neuromuscular effects of manipulation have been expounded, including suggestions of placebo or psychological effect. Undoubtedly, these phenomena do play a part in any "laying on of hands," but further studies to assess physiological effects are indicated.

Numerous techniques are advocated for manipulation. Some are merely gentle mild stretching, termed by some therapists as "mobilization." The most frequently used are techniques intended to achieve the maximum range of passive joint movement, succeeded by a brief "thrust" through the joint for a short distance. Some therapists advocate heat, massage, ultrasound, or ice to precede manipulation, and mobilization with exercise is advocated by others. Still another school feels that rest and immobilization before manipulation gives a better result.

Manipulation is most effective when applied gently and directed specifically and precisely to the segmental joint that is impaired, immobile, or "locked". The technique varies tremendously and is applied in numerous manners according to the theory and concept of manipulation accepted by the practitioner. In the low back, numerous contraindications are self evident such as osteoporosis, the presence of central or peripheral neurological deficits, and the presence of malignancy or fracture. Manipulation should probably never be advocated without adequate X-ray evaluation and interpretation, preceded by a careful neurological examination. Force should always be modified to avoid disruption of tissues such as severe sprain, tearing, subluxation, or dislocation of the joint. Fracture has also been described as resulting from manipulation, as has nerve damage in the vicinity of the manipulated joint.

Exercise

The physiological bases for the use and response to exercises are not all verified. Nevertheless, exercises have been the basis of treatment for low back pain for centuries and at present are still the basic conservative treatment. Before prescribing exercise therapy, it is important to understand normal mechanical function and then to delineate the mechanical dysfunction so that appropriate therapy can be directed to this.

Normally, in the erect stance, the anterior weight-bearing portion of the vertebrae—the intervertebral disks and the taut longitudinal ligaments—maintain functional support of the erect vertebral column without significant assistance of the posterior elements and tissues. Thus, posture and conformity to the center of gravity and alignment are vital in maintaining normal mechanics. Any movement away from the center of gravity initiates muscular action for further support. Leaning forward, either to work or to bend forward, causes the erector spinae muscles to contract immediately to control forward flexion. Initially, this muscular contraction is a subtle isometric one to balance the functional unit. As the spine flexes further forward, the erector muscles gradually elongate to allow smooth flexion. This muscular elongation continues until the spine has flexed approximately 45° forward. At this point, the supraspinous ligament has been fully elongated and stops further flexion. Similarly, the connective tissue of the fascia muscles has also been elongated to its fullest, and further flexion is prevented. Beyond this point, further forward flexion, such as bending to lift or to touch the floor, is accomplished by rotation of the pelvis around the hip joints. This pelvic rotation, now supporting a fully flexed lumbar spine, requires gradual elongation of the posterior thigh and leg muscles to achieve full extension.

Return to a full erect posture requires reversal of these flexion patterns. The pelvis rotates back by virtue of gradual contraction of the posterior thigh and leg muscles until the body has reached 45° of forward flexion. At this point, the functional unit supraspinous ligaments no longer support the spine, and the erector spinae muscles contract isotonically to bring the spine to full erect posture.

These normal patterns can be impaired by disuse, distraction, and misuse as well as by local disease of the spinal tissues themselves. In addition, limitation of motion imposed by inflexibility of nonmuscular tissues can also restrict physiological motion and cause pain.

In acute low back pain, there is usually some protective spasm in which the muscles automatically splint the particular segments or the patient subconsciously chooses not to move that part for fear of inducing further pain. If this action is bilateral, an antalgic spine results, an erect spine with no physiological lordosis and no possible flexion. If spasm is unilateral, scoliosis results.

Exercises are usually prescribed to overcome these functional and painful neuromuscular impairments. They are considered to (a) restore normal flexibility, (b) retrain neurophysiological motor patterns and restore the balance between the agonists and antagonists, (c) develop normal proprioceptive feedback patterns, and (d) promote muscle strength and endurance. These objectives may require extended relearning and, after the initial training, demand the redevelopment of automatic implementation.

The following exercises are normally prescribed to achieve these objectives:

1. Knee-chest exercises are intended to elongate the erector spinae muscles. Done slowly and gently, the exercises can elongate the contracted musculature and connective tissue. When used in conjunction with simultaneous neck flexion, the abdominal flexors also contract and cause reciprocal relaxation of the extensors.

2. Pelvic tilting exercises accomplish the same goals as knee-chest exercises and establish the proprioceptive concept of decreased lumbar lordosis.

3. Abdominal exercises, by contracting the abdominal wall, increase intra-abdominal pressure and thus help to unload interdiskal pressure. They also decrease lumbar lordosis, as well as causing reciprocal relaxation of the erector spinae muscles. Lateral flexion exercises elongate both the small erector and the larger lumbar muscles and the sacrospinatus muscles around the spine.

In summary, the ultimate goal of exercise is proper body mechanics, which incorporates a full range of active and passive movements.

REFERENCES

1. Arroyo, P. (1966): Electromyography in the evaluation of reflex muscle spasm. *J. Fla. Med. Assoc.*, 53:29–31.
2. Bonica, J. J. (1957): Management of myofascial pain syndromes in general practice. *J. A. M. A.*, 164:732–738.
3. Cailliet, R. (1977): *Soft Tissue Pain and Disability*. F. A. Davis & Co., Philadelphia.
4. Cailliet, R. (1980): *Low Back Pain Syndrome*, 3rd ed. F. A. Davis & Co., Philadelphia.
5. Cannon, J. T., and Liebeskind, J. C. (1979): Descending control systems in mechanisms of pain and analgesic compounds. In: *Mechanisms of Pain and Analgesic Compounds*, edited by R. F. Beers and E. G. Bassett, Raven Press, New York.
6. Farfan, H. F. (1973): *Mechanical Disorders of the Low Back*. Lea and Febiger, Philadelphia.
7. Grant, A. E. (1964): Massage with ice in the treatment of painful conditions of the musculoskeletal system. *Arch. Phys. Med Rehabil.*, 45:233–238.
8. Gross, D. (1974): Pain and autonomic nervous system. In: *Advances in Neurology, Vol. 4*, edited by J. J. Bonica, pp. 99–103. Raven Press, New York.
9. Kraus, H. (1941): Use of surface anesthesia in treatment of painful motion. *J. A. M. A.*, 116:2582–2583.
10. Mennell, J. McM. (1960): Back Pain—Diagnosis and Treatment Using Manipulative Therapy. Little, Brown and Co., Boston.
11. Mennell, J. McM. (1975): The therapeutic use of cold. *J. Osteopathic Assoc.*, 74:1146–1158.
12. Melzack, R., Jeans, M. E., Stratford, J. G., and Monks, R. C. (1980): Ice massage and transcutaneous electrical stimulation: Comparison of treatment for low back pain. *Pain*, 9:209–217.
13. Travell, J., and Renzler, S. H. (1952): The myofascial genesis of pain. *Postgrad. Med.*, 11:425–434.

Chronic Low Back Pain, edited by
M. Stanton-Hicks and Robert Boas.
Raven Press, New York © 1982.

Exercise Therapy: The Role of Physical Therapy

Linda Czerniawski

*Department of Physical Therapy, University of Massachusetts Medical Center,
Worcester, Massachusetts 01604*

Managing the patient with chronic low back pain is rarely considered a challenge in the average physical therapy department. The multiplicity of problems encountered in these patients poses the need for a team approach if they are to be treated effectively. However, only in larger medical centers is this approach feasible.

If, in fact, the clinician is providing similar therapy for all "low back" patients—such modalities as heat, massage, and Williams flexion exercises (Fig. 1)—without giving any thought to individual treatment, he can expect a high failure rate. No one treatment routine will cure all patients. It is here, on first referral from the physician, that the challenge arises. Without thorough evaluations of the patient's problem, the opportunity for an appropriate treatment regime is lost. The various physical problems—pain, spasm, decreased function in everyday activities, poor posture, poor muscle strength and flexibility, and obesity—are only compounded by the emotional barriers raised against getting well again. Such factors are decreased self-esteem, distorted body image, anger, health care dependency, and

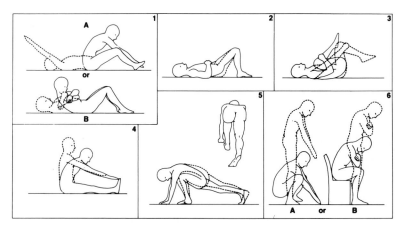

FIG. 1. Postural instructions for Williams flexion exercises. (From Williams, ref. 52, with permission.)

financial compensation. Sternbach (46) describes certain character disturbances in patients with chronic pain that further confound the problem for the therapist who is relatively untrained in the psychology of the disabled. With such overwhelming evidence against recovery by these patients, it is no wonder that the therapist feels "defeated" before the problem is even approached. However, with a systematic approach to the individual problems of each patient, a rehabilitation perspective can be met by any physical therapy department that has a minimum level of equipment and personnel.

WHERE IS YOUR PAIN?
Please mark on the drawings below the areas where you feel your pain.

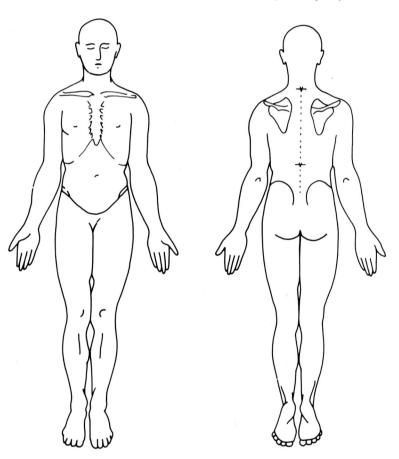

FIG. 2.   Sample pain diagram for completion by patient.

This is not a treatise on any specific exercise program, such as that designed by Williams (52), Brown (9), or Kraus (31), or the New York Hospital program (33). Rather is it an attempt to encourage more innovative thinking and the use of various evaluative skills in approaching the patient with low back pain. Acceptance of the physician's referral must start with a thorough evaluation. Treatment must start with a cause and effect synthesis.

A simple diagnosis of "low back pain" is insufficient. If cause and effect are to be established so that treatment is not a "shot in the dark," both physician and therapist must search for the pain-producing tissue giving rise to the patient's symptoms.

A thorough history of injury, past treatments, and their results is needed to help define the nature of the injury. Many texts provide details as to which aspects are most appropriate in the history (14,21,27,31,33,36,40,51,52) and what weight one should place on the patient's own statement of his pain. A pain diagram (Fig. 2)

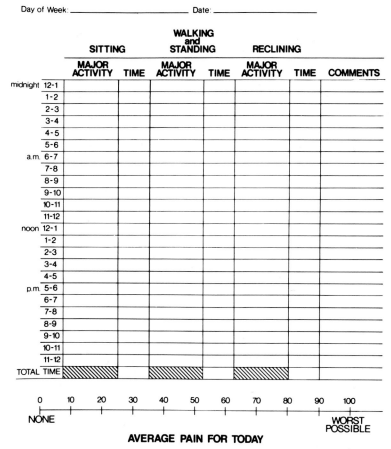

FIG. 3. Activity diary (Based on Sternbach, ref. 46.)

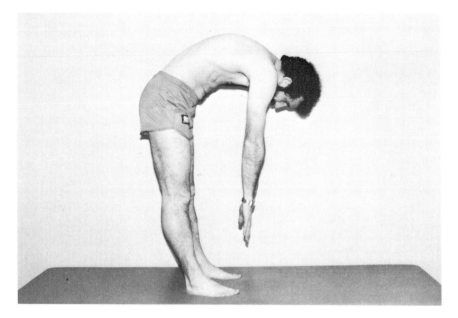

FIG. 4. Patient in forward bend. Distance is measured from fingertips to floor.

may be filled in by the patient on the initial and subsequent visits. It may prove to be useful in localizing symptoms or documenting the changing nature of pain symptomatology. For the patient with chronic pain, an activity diary (Fig. 3) with a pain rating scale provides baseline data on a patient's day-to-day functioning and may then be used to establish an activity program based on existing endurance.

The objective exam is undertaken to reproduce the patient's pain. Again, many texts provide guidelines on the organization and content of the exam (14,21,27,31,33,36,40,51,52). It should be conducted in a manner that provides the examiner with the maximum amount of information and the minimum number of position changes for the patient. Keen observation will reveal whether a patient has been consistent with his complaints and his demonstrated symptomatology.

With the patient erect, gait and posture are evaluated for deviations from midline, asymmetrical muscle bulk, flattened or increased lordosis, and weight distribution (14,29,31,33,40). Watching the patient as he changes clothes or positions may provide the therapist with a relative idea of the severity of the patient's symptoms.

Regional and motion-segment mobility are tested next. It is important that the patient be undressed so that the spine is easily visualized and can be palpated. The range of forward flexion is noted by measuring the distance from fingertips to floor (Fig. 4). The rhythm of movement is noted by palpating the spinous processes and observing the spine for flattened areas in the curve. "Overpressure," a stretch applied by the examiner at the end of active range is applied to check for additional range but is not recommended in the presence of pain and spasm.

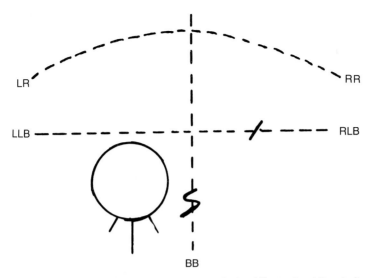

FIG. 5. A method for recording the results of regional spinal mobility testing. LR = Left rotation; LLB = left lateral bend; RR = right rotation; RLB = right lateral bend; BB = backward bend; S = Hypermobility; / = hypomobility. Circle represents vertebra, posterior view.

Extension, lateral flexion, and rotation are actively tested in the same manner. All motions are recorded on a simple graph (Fig. 5) along with any specific abnormalities noted during the exam.

While the patient is standing, he is then asked to squat. This is called the "quick test" because it quickly examines hips, knees, and ankles. If even a bounce at the end of the range does not reproduce symptoms in the hips, knees, or ankles, these joints may be ruled out as contributing to the complaint. However, this test should not be done when there is known pathology in any of these joints.

The lower quarter exam is continued by establishing neurological integrity for L2 through S2. Kendall (29) provides the basis for testing and grading representative muscles. It is necessary to perform this test bilaterally and to be aware of any muscle substitutions during the testing procedure. Throughout the exam, sensory status is noted as well.

After the gastrocnemius is tested while the patient is standing—by having him rise up on his toes at least five times—he is then asked to lie supine. Cord signs (Babinski, clonus) should be tested, as well as ankle dorsiflexors, extensor hallucis longus, peroneals, and hip flexors (psoas). Quadriceps may be tested either supine or prone. Tests of passive flexibility of the low back, iliopsoas, hamstrings, heelcords, and root tension are next evaluated. As MacNab states in *Backache* (36), reproduction of pain with the straight leg does not necessarily indicate root tension because hamstring spasm may be associated with any painful back lesion. However, it is important to note the arc of movement before pain is experienced and to observe whether or not it is increased with ankle dorsiflexion or decreased with knee flexion. The bowstring test may further confirm the presence of root tension. Hip and knee

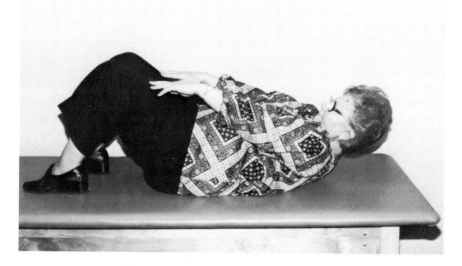

FIG. 6. Patient demonstrating bent knee sit-up.

joint motions and sacroiliac joint tests (14,21,24,27,36,40) are necessary to eliminate these joints as factors contributing to the patient's symptomatology. Finally, the power of the abdominals is tested with a bent knee sit-up (Fig. 6).

With patient lying on his side, the ability to abduct the leg against resistance is tested. Unilateral weakness of the gluteus medius may indeed stress the low back, yet go undetected in gait. Forceful abduction may also point to sacroiliac involvement. The Ober test is a passive measure of tensor fasciae latae flexibility.

With the patient in the prone position, muscle testing is completed by examination of the hamstrings and gluteus maximus. Passive stretch tests include the Ely sign for rectus femoris tightness and the femoral nerve stretch test, which involves slight knee flexion while the hip is being extended. The spine is then palpated for temperature changes, sweating, and tenderness. The therapist who is trained in spinal mobilization may then proceed to evaluate spinal segment mobility (14,21,24,40,41).

Orthopedic manual therapy maintains that joint dysfunction presents as an altered state of mechanics. This may be demonstrated as hypermobility, hypomobility, or an aberrant motion. By testing passive intervertebral motion through palpations between the vertebae, one can grade each segment according to a scale (Table 1); this scale provides the principal indications for treatment (40,41).

The process of correlating the subjective and objective data relating to the patient's history, pain, strength, flexibility, sensation, reflexes, and palpations, is a task that requires an understanding of musculoskeletal pathology and the phenomenon of referred pain. Referred pain is dermatone specific, that is, it can be traced back to a nerve or muscle lesion at the same level. When more specific structures are cited

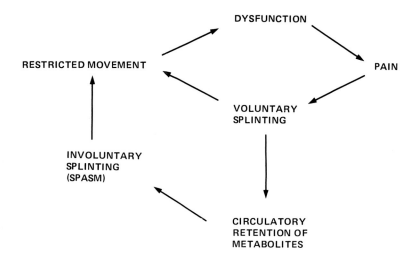

FIG. 7. Involuntary splinting cycle. (From Paris, ref. 41, with permission.)

TABLE 1. *Grading of passive intervertebral motion and indications for treatment*

Grading		Treatment
0–Ankylosed		No treatment
1–Considerable restriction	Hypomobile	Mobilization
2–Slight restriction		Mobilization
3–Normal		No treatment
4–Slight increase in mobility	Hypermobile	No treatment
5–Considerable increase in mobility		Stabilization, exercise, posture, corset
6–Unstable		Surgical intervention

Based on Paris, ref. 41.

as the cause of pain and dysfunction, a more specific treatment program can be provided relative to each patient's needs.

Drs. Loeser, Cailliet, and Raj *(this volume)* stated that chronic low back pain is a different disease entity from acute low back pain. As such, treatment of the two conditions differs frequently, although occasionally there may be some overlap. The initial goal of treatment may be to relieve muscle spasm. Muscle spasm prevents ease of movement and, if present for prolonged periods, is self-perpetuating as lactic acid and other metabolites build up in the muscle tissues due to loss of the normal contraction/relaxation cycle of muscle activity (Fig. 7) (41). Massage, a frequently underused treatment modality, may break the pain cycle. Relaxation of tense muscles allows increased blood flow through the tissues. Although the effects are temporary, the additional range of movement may then allow further treatment techniques to be applied. The typical physical therapy department is also amply provided with the various heat and cold modalities, such as diathermy, ultrasound, whirlpool, hot packs, and ice packs. These modalities are also useful in decreasing muscle spasm and local inflammation, increasing local blood flow, decreasing pain, and providing local and general relaxation (35). They should be used as adjuncts to achieve functional goals.

Mobilization techniques may also decrease pain and muscle splinting (neurophysiological effects). In a hypomobile joint, increasing range of motion is noted (mechanical effect) (41). However, these techniques cannot be learned from textbook pictures and should, therefore, be left to well-trained clinicians.

Another "passive" mode of treatment is the use of transcutaneous electrical nerve stimulation (TENS). Its value in the treatment of chronic low back pain has been limited. However, as a pain-relieving modality, it should not be overlooked. It may very well provide the stimulus needed to start a patient on an activity program.

For the patient's emotional well-being and the restoration of the patient's self-esteem, therapy that goes beyond mere palliation must be initiated as soon as possible. Keeping the patient with chronic low back pain in a passive therapeutic role only reinforces his sick and frail image. The therapist must provide the stimulus that enables the patient to become active in his own health care. Although taken from a book on quadraplegic rehabilitation, the following quotation may apply to any rehabilitation program:

> As strength and endurance increase, there must be a purpose beyond the increase itself, for these qualities reach their peak only as they are harnessed for functional use. The earlier the improvement is related to purposeful activity, the sooner the patient will reach his maximum level of rehabilitation (17).

Patient education and involvement are essential to any successful treatment program. A recent growth in the number of "Back Schools" has provided the opportunity to therapists to teach patients more effective ways of both protecting their backs

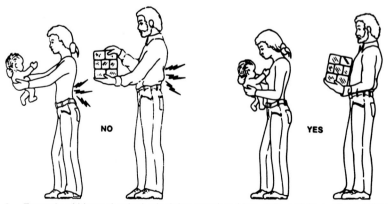

FIG. 8. Example of biomechanical principles translated into daily activities. (From White, ref. 51, with permission.)

and managing their back pain (3,5,23,26). If a patient understands more about his own anatomy and the biomechanical functioning of his spine, he may more readily adapt this knowledge to all aspects of his everyday life. *Clinical Biomechanics of the Spine* by White and Panjabi (51) provides the most comprehensive review of the literature to date on spine function and dysfunction. Many biomechanical aspects are translated into the "why's and wherefore's" of daily activity (Fig. 8).

Exercise for the patient with chronic low back pain remains the one issue of controversy, and unfortunately, the literature is devoid of clinical trials proving or disproving the effectiveness of one form of exercise over another. In Taylor's study of the physiological effects of bed rest (49), he states that "the fundamental components of fitness are coordination, speed, strength and endurance," and that "physical conditioning is always the result of activity, i.e., muscular excercise." When his normal subjects were placed on strict bed rest for 3 weeks, cardiovascular response to erect posture did not return to normal for over 7 weeks. Endurance basically reflects cardiovascular function, and it is this deterioration that underlies the whole deconditioning process. Other studies have been done that further corroborate the deleterious effects of enforced bed rest (8). Tabary's study (48) further shows that immobilization, especially where the range is shortened, may actually decrease the number of sarcomeres in series within a muscle fiber by up to 40%, thus changing the length-tension property that manifests itself as a considerable decrease in extensibility. In view of all of these findings, it is no wonder that the patient with chronic low back pain, especially the one who has enforced his own bed rest routine, suffers from increased pain upon trying to resume activity with exercise. His own mechanical and emotional problems are only compounded by these deconditioning factors.

In order to reverse these processes, a progressive conditioning program that will adapt to the strength, flexibility, and endurance baseline of the patient is necessary. When starting such a program, the therapist must keep in mind three general rules that are invaluable in modifying exercise and activity for the patient with chronic low back pain.

1. Exercises must be smooth and rhythmical, so that they do not subject muscles and joints to sudden unexpected stresses and strains. Muscle contraction should be followed by relaxation to allow normal circulatory conditions to be restored in the muscle before its next contraction.

2. Exercise must be based on sound starting positions. To strengthen weak muscles or mobilize stiff joints, the starting positions of the exercises should be as steady as possible so as to give the working muscles a firm origin from which to work, and the level of difficulty should be increased gradually.

3. Exercises must provide a smooth progression from the stage of extreme weakness to the stage of full use, against the stresses of normal working conditions. In addition, all exercises that aim at strengthening weak muscles should provide as wide a range of movement as possible (13). In the patient with chronic low back pain, starting an exercise in the pain-free arc of movement may prove useful for building toward a freer movement.

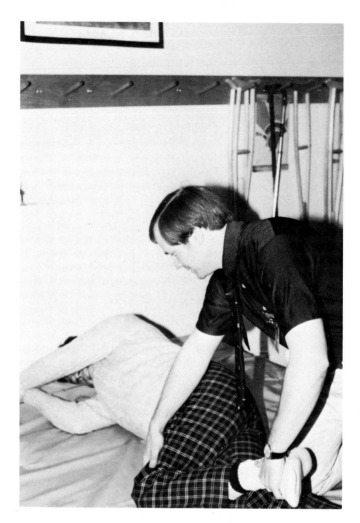

FIG. 9. Therapist assisting patient in segmental rolling on mat.

When evaluation of the patient points to the need to strengthen or stretch any particular muscle group, the steadfast use of only one approach (e.g., William's flexion) is simply to ignore all evaluation criteria. There are many options available to the therapist to create exercise programs, some based on traditional modes of thought, some not so traditional. But no rule says that the patient with low back pain must exercise while lying on his back. A developmental approach to movement, based on the theories of Kabat or Rood or Bobath (7) is not restricted to use with neurological patients. A "mat" program of this nature frequently utilizes activities and postures normally assumed by the patient in his activities of daily living. Rolling

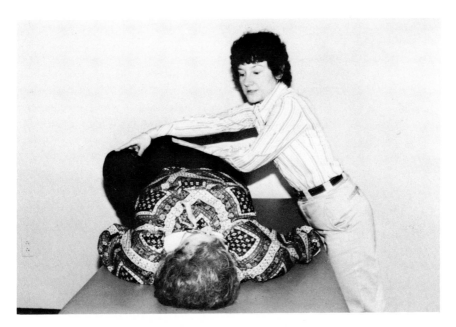

FIG. 10. Patient working on rhythmic stabilization activities.

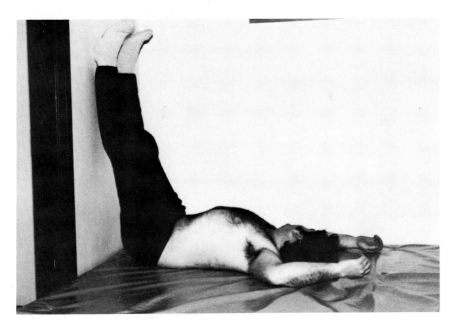

FIG. 11. Patient maintaining prolonged stretch of hamstrings.

in bed all too often becomes a superhuman effort when pain prevents segmental motion (Fig. 9).

The literature continues to support the importance of strengthening the abdominal muscles. Farfan reports that the abdominal muscles, in combination with the back extensors, minimize dangerous torque and shear stresses in the lumbar spine during a lift (19). However, in the presence of erector spinae spasm, the phenomenon of reciprocal inhibition takes place and there is no tension in opposing muscles (44). Muscular re-education of the abdominal muscles may be necessary in chronic cases. A rational progression of abdominal strengthening must be accompanied by a reduction in the spasm of the opposing group of muscles.

Trunk and hip extensor strengthening is approached by using sound neurophysiological principles. Working the trunk extensors in a shortened range, such as in a "pivotprone" position, biases the gamma motor system so that the muscle spindle is more receptive to postural stretch. Then, having the patient assume the quadruped position stretches the low back and gluteals. This will facilitate abdominals and hip flexors for co-contraction, which is a balance of muscular tone around a joint, and

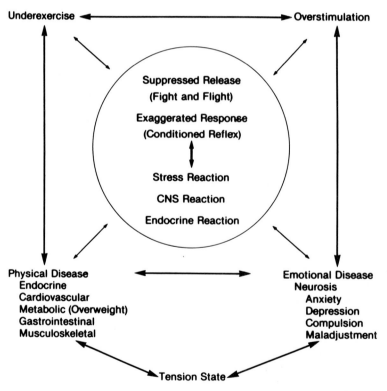

FIG. 12. Diagram of forces acting on the typical urban person, who is overrested, overfed, overstressed, underexercised, and underreleased. (From Kraus, ref. 31, with permission.)

will provide a stable base permitting movement to occur in any direction (7). These principles may be applied to any developmental or functional position (Fig. 10). This allows for more general body conditioning as opposed to isolated isotonic muscle strengthening. Here a balance exists between eccentric, concentric, and isometric contractions.

One of the more difficult tasks posed for the patient with low back pain is the stretching of his shortened hamstrings. As a multi-arthrodial muscle, its function is phasic in nature. The hamstrings are mainly "mobilizers" rather than "stabilizers." A quick stretch will facilitate rather than inhibit the muscle, due to the muscle spindle. Ia afferents signal velocity of stretch; II afferents signal length of stretch. With prolonged positioning of the phasic muscle, the receptor activity of Ia and II gradually diminishes and muscle inhibition occurs. Table 2 compares the muscle spindle afferents of phasic muscles to the tonic muscles and describes the nature of their response to prolonged stretch. Therefore, a maintained stretch of more than 20 min is recommended to overcome the facilitatory effect of stretching the hamstrings (Fig. 11).

Whereas the traditional approach to physical problems through exercise is the province of the physical therapist, an increasing interest in "holistic" and nontraditional therapies is developing. The patient with painful spasm can obtain relief by means of massage, etc. Education in basic ergonomic principles, correction of gait and posture, mobilization where appropriate, and attention to the environment are also generic to the present epidemic of low back pain. However, there are still "suppressed release," stress reactions that remain unexpressed. Kraus depicts this as a lifelong battle between ourselves and the environment (Fig. 12) (31).

To meet this need for stress reduction in the patient with chronic pain, more physical therapy departments are developing programs aimed at teaching relaxation. The techniques of self-hypnosis, transcendental meditation, the "relaxation response," biofeedback and many other relaxation techniques are used to break into

TABLE 2. *Muscle spindle afferents: response to stretch*

| Muscle type | Type of afferent fiber | | Effect of prolonged stretch |
	Ia	II	
Phasics-	(+) Muscle stretched	(+) Flexor	Ia adapts quickly; II adapts slowly.
Mobilizers	(−) Antagonist	(−)Extensor	After 20 min. input from stretch receptors is reduced.
Tonics-	(+) Muscle stretched	(+) Flexor	Ia adapt; II inhibitory.
Stabilizers	(−) Antagonist	(−) Extensor	The effective period for inhibition of tonic postural extensors is the first 20 min.

+ = facilitate; − = inhibit.

the tension-disease cycle. This can become a stepping stone for decreasing the patient's dependence on the health-care system and fostering a self-reliance on innate strength. Preliminary results of the Stress Reduction and Relaxation program at the University of Massachusetts Medical Center have substantiated the innate strength that exists when a deliberate attempt is made to unite mind and body. This pilot program conducted by Dr. Jon Kabat-Zinn was developed around groups of 10 to 15 patients who suffered from chronic pain and/or high stress diseases such as hypertension. Patients are taught "awareness" meditation—a Zen practice—which they are required to practice daily for 10 weeks. There is a weekly 2-hr session for yoga-like exercise, meditation, and group discussion. Unpublished results already indicate a significant reduction in pain and/or other stress symptoms, together with an increase in social and functional activity.

The end result of therapy should be that the patient achieves the maximum possible function within the limitations of his or her environment, with lowered dependency on drugs and bed rest. There is also a need to encourage recreational and sports activity to mobilize the patient, and once the patient has reached the optimal level of activity, to sustain it at the same level. There is much to be said about putting "fun" into the rehabilitation scheme. A World Health Organization study, *Habitual Physical Activity and Health* (2), positively correlates sports and recreation (walking, running, swimming, gardening, and hunting) with physical fitness. Certainly, it is of benefit to recommend nontorsional sports to the patient with chronic low back pain so that maintenance of activity does not become a chore.

REFERENCES

1. Anderson, B. J. G., Ortengren, R., Nachemson, A., Elfstrom, G., and Broman, H. (1975): The sitting posture: an electromyographic and discometric study. *Orthop. Clin. N. Am.*, 6:105–120.
2. Anderson, K. L., Masiron, R., Rutenfranz, J., and Selinger, V. (1978): *Habitual Physical Activity and Health*. World Health Organization, Copenhagen.
3. Attix, E. A., and Tate, M. A. (1979): Low Back School: A conservative method for the treatment of low back pain. *J. Miss. State Med. Assoc.*, 20:4–9.
4. Basmajian, J. V., editor (1978): *Therapeutic Exercise*. The Williams & Wilkins Co., Baltimore, Maryland.
5. Bergquist-Ullman, M., and Larsson, V. (1977): Acute low back pain in industry. A controlled prospective study with special reference to therapy and confounding factors. *Acta Orthop. Scand.*, 170:1–117.
6. Boulton-Davies, I. M. (1979): Physiotherapists–Teachers of the public. *Physiotherapy*, 65:280.
7. Bouman, H. D., editor (1967): An exploratory and analytical survey of therapeutic exercise: Northwestern University Special Therapeutic Exercise Project. *Am. J. Phys. Med.*, 46.
8. Brannon, E. W., Rockwood, C. A., and Potts, P. (1963): The influence of specific exercises in the prevention of debilitating musculoskeletal disorders; implications in physiological conditioning for prolonged weightlessness. *Aero. Med.*, 34:900–906.
9. Brown, I. (1970): Intensive exercises for the low back. *Phys. Ther.*, 50:487–498.
10. Burkart, S. L., and Beresford, W. A. (1979): The aging intervertebral disk. *Phys. Ther.*, 59:969–970.
11. Carmichael, S. W., and Burkart, S. L. (1979): Clinical anatomy of the lumbosacral complex. *Phys. Ther.*, 59:966–968.
12. Chadwick, P. R. (1979): Advising patients on back care. *Physiotherapy*, 65:277–278.
13. Colson, J. (1969): *Progressive exercise therapy in rehabilitation and physical education*. The Williams & Wilkins Co., Baltimore, Maryland.

14. Cyraix, J. (1971): *Textbook of Orthopaedic Medicine*. Vols. I & II. The Williams & Wilkins Co., Baltimore, Maryland.
15. Edgar, M. (1979): Pathologies associated with lifting. *Physiotherapy*, 65:245–247.
16. Edgelow, P. I. (1979): Physical examination of the lumbosacral complex. *Phys. Ther.*, 59:974–977.
17. Etter, M. F. (1968): *Exercise for the prone patient*. Wayne State University Press, Detroit, Michigan.
18. Evans, D. P.. Burke, M. S., Lloyd, K. N., Roberts, E. E., and Roberts, G. M. (1978): Lumbar spinal manipulation on trial. Part I—Clinical Assessment. *Rheumatol. Rehabil.*, 17:46–53.
19. Farfan, H. F. (1975): Muscular mechanism of the lumbar spine and the position of power and efficiency. *Orthop. Clin. N. Am.*, 6:135–144.
20. Farfan, H. F. (1978): The biomechanical advantage of lordosis and hip extension for upright activity: man as compared with other anthropoids. *Spine*, 3:336–342.
21. Fisk, J. W. (1977): *A Practical Guide to Management of the Painful Neck and Back; Diagnosis, Manipulation, Exercises, Prevention*. Charles C Thomas Publishers, Springfield, Illinois.
22. Fisk, J. W. (1979): The passive hamstring stretch test: clinical evaluation. *NZ Med. J.*, 89:209–211.
23. Gottlieb, H. J., Alperson, B. L., Koller, R., and Hockersmith, V. (1979): An innovative program for the restoration of patients with chronic back pain. *Phys. Ther.*, 59:996–999.
24. Grieve, G. P. (1976): The sacroiliac joint. *Physiotherapy*, 62:384–400.
25. Grillner, S., Nilsson, J., and Thorstensson, A. (1978): Intra-abdominal pressure changes during natural movements in man. *Acta Physiol. Scand.*, 103:275–283.
26. Grimes, D., Bennion, D., Blush, K., and Duncan, M. E. (1980): Back School—Teaching Patients to Love Their Backs. *Res. Staff Phys.*, 26:60–68.
27. Hoppenfeld, S. (1976): *Physical Examination of the Spine and Extremities*. Appleton-Century-Crofts, New York.
28. Jayson, M., editor (1976): *The Lumbar Spine and Back Pain*. Grune & Stratton, New York.
29. Kendall, H. O., Kendall, F. P., Wadsworth, G. E. (1971): *Muscles–Testing and Function*. The Williams & Wilkins Co., Baltimore, Maryland.
30. Kessler, R. M. (1979): Acute Symptomatic Disk Prolapse: Clinical Manifestations and Therapeutic Considerations. *Phys. Ther.*, 59:978–987.
31. Kraus, H. (1970): *Clinical Treatment of Back and Neck Pain*. McGraw-Hill Book Co., New York.
32. Kulak, R., Schultz, A., Belytschko, T., Galante, J. (1975): Biomechanical characteristics of vertebral motion segments and intervertebral discs. *Orthop. Clin. N. Am.*, 6:121–133.
33. LaFreniere, J. G. (1979): *The Low Back Patients: Procedures for Treatment by Physical Therapy*. Masson Publishing U.S.A., Inc., New York.
34. Lamb, D. W. (1979): The Neurology of Spinal Pain. *Phys. Ther.*, 59:971–973.
35. Licht, S., editor (1965): *Therapeutic Heat and Cold*. Elizabeth Licht, Publisher, New Haven, Connecticut.
36. MacNab, I. (1977): *Backache*. The Williams & Wilkins Co., Baltimore, Maryland.
37. McKenzie, R. A. (1979): Prophylaxis in recurrent low back pain. *NZ Med. J.*, 89:22–23.
38. Mooney, V. (1979): Surgery and postsurgical management of the patient with low back pain. *Phys. Ther.*, 59:1000–1006.
39. Nielsen, A. J. (1978): Spray and stretch for myofascial pain. *Phys. Ther.*, 58:567–569.
40. Paris, S. V. (1979): The Spine, etiology and treatment of dysfunction, including joint manipulation. Course notes (revised). Institute of Graduate Health Sciences, Atlanta, Ga.
41. Paris, S. V. (1979): Mobilization of the Spine. *Phys. Ther.*, 59:988–995.
42. Roberts, G. M., Roberts, E. E., Lloyd, K. N., Burke, M. S., and Evans, D. P. (1978): Lumbar spinal manipulation on trial. Part II–radiological assessment. *Rheumatol. Rehabil.*, 17:54–59.
43. Seres, J., Newman, R. (1976): Results of treatment of chronic low back pain at the Portland Pain Center. *J. Neurosurg.*, 45:32–36.
44. Sherrington, C. (1911): *The Integrative Action of the Nervous System*, pp. 150–170. Yale University Press, New Haven, Connecticut.
45. Sims-Williams, H., Jayson, M. I., Young, S. M., Baddeley, H., and Collins, E. (1978): Controlled trial of mobilization and manipulation for patients with low back pain in general practice. *Br. Med. J.*, 2:1338–1340.
46. Sternbach, R. A. (1974): *Pain Patients: Traits and Treatment*. Academic Press, Inc., New York.
47. Strachan, A. (1979): Back care in industry. *Physiotherapy*, 65:249–251.
48. Tabary, J. C., Tabary, C., Tardieu, G., and Goldspink, G. (1972): Physiological and structural changes in the cat's soleus muscle due to immobilization at different lengths by plaster casts. *J. Physiol. (Lond.)*, 224:231–244.

49. Taylor, H. L. (1951): Physiological effects of bed rest and immobilization. In: *Physical Medicine and Rehabilitation for the Clinician*, edited by F. Krusen. W. B. Saunders Co., Philadelphia, Pennsylvania.
50. Troup, J. D. (1979): Biomechanics of the vertebral column. Its application to prevention of back pain in the population and to assessment of working capacity in working patients with lumbar spinal disability. *Physiotherapy*, 65:238–244.
51. White, A. A., and Panjabi, M. M. (1978): *Clinical Biomechanics of the Spine*. J. B. Lippincott Co., New York.
52. Williams, P. C. (1965): *The Lumbosacral Spine*. McGraw-Hill Book Co., New York.

Chronic Low Back Pain, edited by
M. Stanton-Hicks and Robert Boas.
Raven Press, New York © 1982.

Epidural Steroid Therapy for Low Back Pain

*Harold Carron and **Timothy C. Toomey

*Department of Anesthesiology, School of Medicine, University of Virginia,
Charlottesville, Virginia 22908; and **Pain Clinic, Dental Research Unit, Bldg. 210H,
University of North Carolina Dental School, Chapel Hill, North Carolina 27514

Early attempts at relief of low back pain utilized injections of large volumes of saline or local anesthetic mixtures via the caudal-epidural route (7). The report by Lindhal and Rexed (9) that both inflammation and compression of a nerve root are necessary for the production of pain prompted the suggestion that bathing the pathologically inflamed and compressed nerve root with a local anesthetic containing a corticosteroid could reduce the swelling and inflammation responsible for the pain.

Seghal and Gardner (10) reported on a large series of patients with epidural adhesions who were benefited by epidural and intrathecal steroid block. Fishman and Christy (6), Ito (8), and Swerdlow and co-workers (11) also utilized steroid injections for various back pain disorders, introducing the corticosteroids at segmental levels into either the epidural or subarachnoid space.

CLINICAL INDICATIONS

Since most reports of extradural corticosteroid injections for sciatica have been enthusiastic (5,8,11,13), the technique has been extended to the treatment of low back pain of multiple etiologies, often with equivocal results. Temporary improvement may occur in the presence of nerve root irritation due to spondylolisthesis, osteoarthritis, or trauma involving the posterior primary rami of the spinal nerve roots. In these disorders, epidural steroid therapy may provide symptomatic relief that is sufficient to permit the institution of exercise programs, back care education, the fitting of orthotic devices, and other therapeutic measures. However, when a single block does not provide the desired response, alternative therapy should be considered.

The most effective use of epidural corticosteroid therapy is for the treatment of nerve root entrapment and irritation secondary to discogenic disease. Symptomatically, discogenic disease is characterized by radicular pain over dermatomal distribution, with reproducible sensory deficits over the area supplied by the particular nerve root, and an increase in radicular pain with coughing, sneezing, straining at stool, or acute flexion of the trunk. The pain is also increased with prolonged sitting or standing and relieved by rest in the supine position.

193

Positive physical signs of appropriate sensory deficits, motor weakness, muscle atrophy or fibrillation, depressed or absent reflexes, sciatic notch tenderness, and increase in radicular pain with foot flexion or head lift during straight leg raising confirm the presence of an entrapped and inflamed nerve root.

TECHNIQUE OF EPIDURAL INJECTION

Every patient with low back pain and sciatica, except those developing bladder and bowel dysfunction, should be placed on a trial of at least 2 weeks of anti-inflammatory analgesics and absolute bed rest prior to institution of any type of invasive therapy. When this program proves ineffectual in decreasing the symptoms, a rational plan for sequential therapy should be developed. The figure suggests a protocol for the management of low back pain that is conservative in approach but definitive in therapy.

Epidural steroid injection should be performed following failure of enforced bed rest. Winnie (13) and others claim improved results with subarachnoid over epidural injection. However, Abram (1) performed subarachnoid steroid injections on patients with low back pain who had failed to obtain improvement with epidural steroids. He concluded that there was no significant difference in results in this group following subarachnoid steroid administration. Since the nerve root compression in discogenic disease is extradural, it appears rational to introduce the steroid epidurally at the site of compression rather than subarachnoid where it would be subject to dilution and dispersion. Therefore, epidural puncture should be done at the site of nerve root entrapment, one level above that of emergence of the affected root, with the patient in the lateral decubitus position and the painful side recumbent.

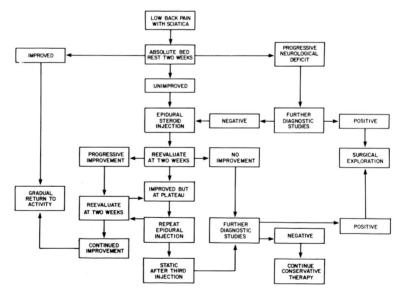

FIG. 1.   Sequential therapy for low back pain and sciatica.

When the epidural space has been identified by loss of resistance or hanging drop techniques, 80 mg (2 ml) of methylprednisolone acetate (Depo-Medrol®) or 50 mg (2 ml) of triamcinolone diacetate (Aristocort Intralesional®) are suspended in 4 to 6 ml of a sensory-blocking concentration of local anesthetic and, after negative aspiration for blood or spinal fluid, slowly injected into the epidural space. In patients who have previously undergone back surgery, identification of the epidural space may be difficult. Under these circumstances, 2 ml of local anesthetic should be introduced first. With evidence that the anesthetic was placed epidurally (pain relief, segmental sensory loss), this may then be followed by injection of the corticosteroid. Should accidental penetration of the dura occur, this two-part technique will identify introduction of the local anesthetic into the subarachnoid space and permit withdrawal of the needle into the epidural space prior to injection of the corticosteroid.

Following epidural steroid injection, the patient is kept in the lateral position for 10 to 15 minutes to contain the spread of drug to the involved side. Some physicians advocate that sciatic stretch exercises be initiated and continued over a period of weeks to prevent development or recurrence of perineural adhesions, although there is no evidence either that stretching or injection break down adhesions or that steroids prevent their formation.

As shown in the figure, 2 weeks after epidural block, the patient should be reevaluated for changes in symptoms and physical signs. If there is progressive improvement in pain and function, no further treatment is indicated and the patient is reevaluated 2 weeks later for further progress. However, if after the first injection physical symptoms and signs initially showed improvement but then reached a plateau of progress, the therapy should be repeated and the patient again reevaluated after another 2-week interval. Rarely should more than a total of three epidural blocks be performed.

If at 2 weeks after the initial injection, the patient's signs and symptoms are unchanged or worse, block therapy is abandoned and additional investigative procedures are instituted (electromyography, contrast myelography, epidural venography) to better define the pathology. The presence of an intervertebral disk extruded into the spinal canal, the occurrence of bladder or bowel dysfunction, or the progression of neurological deficits is an indication for prompt surgical exploration.

COMPLICATIONS

Although epidural corticosteroid injection is a popular and relatively complication-free procedure, there are inherent risks involved in the procedure. These include corticosteroid toxicity with mental confusion, fluid retention, Cushingoid facies, and other evidence of steroid excess or later, adrenal suppression. The risks of local anesthetics include high block with respiratory and circulatory depression, local anesthetic toxicity, accidental subarachnoid injection, prolonged block in patients with demyelinating disease, and infection with local abscess formation.

Little information is available on the long-term effects of epidurally placed steroids on neural tissue. Delaney et al. (4) performed a series of experiments on cats to determine the effect of epidurally injected triamcinolone diacetate in vehicle and of the vehicle itself on the peripheral nerve roots, root sleeves, and meninges. Examination by light and electron microscopy showed no evidence of acute or chronic neural toxicity in these animals, suggesting that epidural administration of local anesthetic and corticosteroid triamcinolone diacetate is a safe procedure. These results, however, cannot be extrapolated to other steroid preparations or to a sequence of epidural injections in any one individual.

RESULTS

Various groups have reported statistics indicating that epidural steroid injections are of value in relieving the symptoms and decreasing the disability of low back pain and sciatica (1,3,4,7,10,13). Comparison of the results of various series of patients treated with epidural steroids is difficult because of differences in criteria for inclusion in any category of improvement. Winnie (13) reported subjective complete relief of symptoms in 80% of patients with either epidural or subarachnoid injections in a small series. Brown reported "excellent to good" results in 100% of patients with acute discogenic disease of less than 3 months duration, but in only 14% of those with pain that had lasted more than 3 months. McLaughlin and co-workers (*personal communication*) reviewed 155 patients 12 to 18 months following treatment with epidural and subarachnoid steroids, dividing the series into those with acute disk herniation unresponsive to conservative treatment and those who suffered from more chronic pain problems. Of this group, 31% were diagnosed as having acute herniated disk disease and 47% as failed laminectomy, or persistence of symptoms despite surgery. The remainder of the group included patients with spondylolisthesis, degenerative changes, and undiagnosed maladies.

As shown in the table, post-treatment results defined patients with "good results" as those who returned to a former level of activity without analgesic medication and those with "poor results" as all others. Six of the "poor result" acute herniated disk group were identified as suffering from an extruded disk in the spinal canal

TABLE 1. *Treatment results (McLaughlin Study)[a]*

Condition	No. of patients (%)
Acute herniated disk	31 patients
Good results	67%
Poor results	33%
Failed laminectomy	78 patients
Good results	33%
Poor results	67%

[a]R. McLaughlin, *personal communication.* Table adapted from H. Carron (1977): Options in therapy for low back pain. *Medical Times*, 105:67–73.

by the persistence of radicular pain with 90° straight leg raising in the presence of an otherwise effective analgesic block.

Arnhoff and co-workers (2) performed a retrospective study on a series of out-patients treated with epidural and subarachnoid steroid therapy for low back pain and sciatica. A questionnaire was sent to each patient 2 years after completion of pain clinic treatment. Results of that survey indicated a significant reduction in pain intensity and frequency, increased ability to walk, bend, and work, and a decrease in time spent in pain-aversive behavior.

There are few long-term follow-up studies of treatment programs for patients with chronic pain, particularly those with low back pain. Those that have been done rarely extended beyond 3 years and were based on costly inpatient treatment models.

Toomey and his colleagues (12) extended the study performed by Arnhoff by an additional 3 years to investigate whether the pain in this group of patients improved, stabilized, or deteriorated as a consequence of elapsed time following corticosteroid therapy. This 5-year study revealed that gains noted 1 to 2 years after treatment were maintained 5 to 6 years later, although there was little change with time in improvement following initial success. This suggests that overall improvement in most areas does not continue progressively over time but occurs soon after treatment.

The study also concerned itself with the integrated pain clinic approach to treatment in which specific therapeutic interventions were only a portion of the overall patient care. The long-term efficacy of pain clinic intervention in the management of chronic pain was confirmed. Subjective ratings of improvement, low percentage of further surgical intervention, and enhanced ability to work that was seen in well over half the patients are supportive of this. This finding of minimal surgical intervention after treatment emphasized the cost-effectiveness of the outpatient model of pain treatment.

The study revealed that gender-related differences in response to pain clinic treatment are to be expected, with females generally reporting initially a greater intensity of pain than males. Females may be expected to report greater improvement with treatment than males on a wide spectrum of functional abilities. Males tend to be particularly conservative in reporting improvement on the most and least essential functions, perhaps reflecting their more intense need to bolster attitudes and behaviors related to the sick role.

As noted in the study by Arnhoff et al., there are multiple criteria for improvement, and the study by Toomey's group suggests that perceptions related to pain and its interference with significant life functions are central determinants of improvement. Specifically, the subjective variable of experienced pain and the more behavioral variables of time spent in bed and return to work were the most reliable predictors of improvement. Global assessment of improvement may bear little relation to more objective criteria, emphasizing the importance of specific functional ratings of improvement. Toomey concludes that for the majority of patients with chronic low back pain, the outcome may be appreciably affected by the administration of epidural or subarachnoid corticosteroids.

SUMMARY

The injection of epidural steroids to treat chronic low back pain and sciatica is a safe and effective procedure. It should be used in the overall context of managing low back pain and not as the sole therapeutic modality. Although this treatment may be of temporary value in a large group of patients with multiple etiological causes for back pain, it is most effective in treating those patients with positive evidence of nerve root irritation presenting with symptoms that would ordinarily lead to surgical intervention. The use of epidural corticosteroid injections may provide a potent therapeutic alternative to low back surgery and thus prevent the chronic disability that frequently follows exploratory laminectomy and diskectomy.

REFERENCES

1. Abram, S. E. (1978): Subarachnoid corticosteroid injection following inadequate response to epidural steroids for sciatica. *Anesth. Analg. (Cleve.),* 57:313–315.
2. Arnhoff, F. N., Triplett, H. B., and Pokorney, B. (1977): Follow-up status of patients treated with nerve blocks for low back pain. *Anesthesiology,* 46:170–178.
3. Brown, F. W. (1977): Management of diskogenic pain using epidural and intrathecal steroids. *Clin. Orthop.,* 129:72–78.
4. Delaney, T. J., Rowlingson, J. C., Carron, H., and Butler, A. B. (1980): The effects of steroids on nerves and meninges. *Anesth. Analg. (Cleve.),* 59:610–614.
5. Dilke, T. F. W., Burry, H. C., and Graham, R. (1973): Extradural corticosteroid injection in management of lumbar nerve root compression. *Br. Med. J.,* 2:635–637.
6. Fishman, P. A., and Christy, N. P. (1965): Fate of adrenal cortical steroids following intrathecal injection. *Neurology,* 15:1–6.
7. Goebert, H. W., Jallo, S. J., Gardner, W. J., et al. (1960): Sciatica: Treatment with epidural injections of procaine and hydrocortisone. *Cleve. Clin. Q.,* 27:191–197.
8. Ito, R. (1971): The treatment of low back pain and sciatica with corticosteroid injection and its pathophysiological basis. *Univ. Jpn. Orthop. Assoc.,* 45:769–777.
9. Lindhal, O., and Rexed, B. (1951): Histological changes in the spinal nerve roots of operated cases of sciatica. *Acta Orthop. Scand.,* 20:215.
10. Sehgal, A. D., and Gardner, W. J. (1963): Place of intrathecal methylprednisolone acetate in neurological disorders. *Trans. Am. Neurol. Assoc.,* 88:275–276.
11. Swerdlow, M., and Sayle-Creer, W. (1970): The use of extradural injections in the relief of lumbo-sciatic pain. *Anaesthesia,* 25:128.
12. Toomey, T. C., Taylor, A. G., Skelton, M. A., and Carron, H. (1982):Five-year follow-up status of chronic low back pain patients. *Pain (in press).*
13. Winnie, A. P., Hartman, J. T., Meyers, H. L., et al. (1972): Pain Clinic II: Intradural and extradural corticosteroids for sciatica. *Anesth. Analg. (Cleve.),* 51:990–999.

Chronic Low Back Pain, edited by
M. Stanton-Hicks and Robert Boas.
Raven Press,
New York © 1982.

Facet Joint Injections

Robert A. Boas

*Department of Pharmacology and Clinical Pharmacology, School of Medicine,
University of Auckland, New Zealand*

Vertebral facet joint injection, also known as facet denervation, rhizotomy, and rhizolysis, is one of the newer therapies for low back pain. Already, an enthusiastic group of exponents has claimed this as one of the more effective treatments, even for patients with persistent mechanical low back pain that is refractory to other therapies. These reports of success, together with the seemingly rational basis for this therapeutic approach and the emphasis on finding nonsurgical modalities to treat low back pain, have given facet joint injection an unusually rapid acceptance. Whether this approach will withstand the challenge of long-term follow-up and controlled study is still unknown.

Credit for advancing the concept of joint denervation as a therapy rests with W. E. S. Rees (10), who advocated a surgical approach to severence of the posterior sensory nerve. Subsequent dissections by Bradley (3) and Edgar and Ghadially (4) established the anatomy of dorsal facet innervation more precisely and thus paved the way for the more accurate and simpler percutaneous denervation technique later described by Shealy (12). At the same time, a better understanding of the natural history and pathophysiology of degenerative vertebral disorders developed, exemplified particularly in the book by Macnab (7). This understanding focused attention on changes in posterior elements of the spine as a major cause of disordered mechanics and low back pain, thus directing therapeutic emphasis away from intervertebral disk disease as the dominant correctable defect in low back pain.

ANATOMY OF NERVE SUPPLY TO FACET JOINTS

Each of the posterior interlaminar facet or zygoapophyseal joints receives its nerve supply from two branches of the posterior primary ramus that is located at each segmental level. One branch arises from the nerve at the same level as the joint and the other from the segmental level above (Fig. 1). Thus, the L3/4 posterior facets are supplied from sensory branches that are derived from the L3 and L2 segmental nerves on either side, each of these branches passing respectively to the lower and upper poles of the joint. In addition, it is apparent that each segmental nerve supplies two facet joints, one branch going to the lower pole of the facet joint at the same spinal level and the other to the upper pole of the joint below. Further sensory innervation to the muscle, interspinous ligaments, and skin is

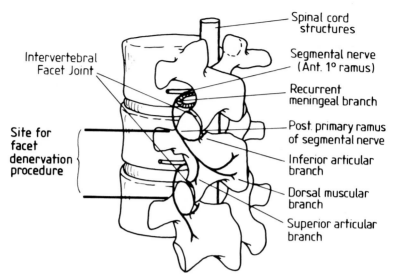

FIG. 1. Segmental innervation of vertebral facet joints. Superior and inferior articular branches from adjacent segmental nerves supply each facet joint. The positions for needle placement to attain denervation at one joint level are shown.

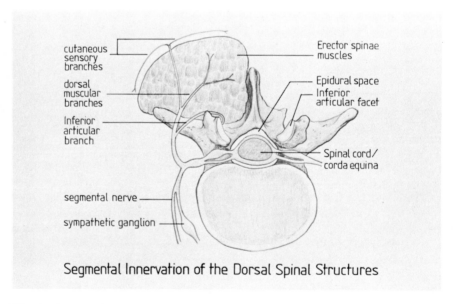

FIG. 2. Segmental innervation of the dorsal spinal structures. The posterior primary ramus of the segmental nerve innervates all posterior elements and integuments in each functional spinal segment. Identification of a precise pain source is made difficult by the compactness and functional interrelationships of these structures.

derived from the same posterior segmental nerve; in this case also, the nerve supplies structures below the spinal segment from which the nerve itself is derived. Stated in yet another way, each joint has dual segmental innervation, and each segmental nerve supplies two facet joints as well as the soft tissues overlying the joints (Fig. 2).

It has still not been elucidated if the joint receives any innervation from within the spinal canal via the recurrent meningeal branch from the posterior ramus (n. Luschka).

The caudad migration of posterior sensory innervation that is evident from the distribution of both the posterior and anterior rami helps to explain distribution of referred pains in the syndrome of facet joint irritation, with distal reference up to two segments below the level of the joint irritation (Fig. 3).

One site for therapeutic intervention of the segmental nerve supply is at the junction of the transverse and articular processes of the dorsal arch. At this level, the bony landmarks are consistent, easily reached percutaneously, and readily identified by X-ray. In addition, there are no vital structures at this level, since the segmental nerve and blood vessels are 1.5 cm away in a more cephalad and ventral plane.

Because of the duality of segmental innervation, each joint must be denervated at two segmental levels—both *at* and *above* the level of the involved joint or capsule (see Fig. 1).

PATHOPHYSIOLOGY OF FACET IRRITATION

A simplistic concept of the pathology of degenerative vertebral disease has been adopted for this presentation (Fig. 4), although it is not the invariable cause for facet pain. In some instances, no skeletal change is evident when joint capsular irritation arises from excessive movement, local trauma, or early changes in which bony and functional disruption are harder to identify. More frequently, however, in the chronic phase of disease, there is a discernible pattern of changes.

The common initiating disorder is a reduction in intervertebral disk space following disk disease, as the result of age, trauma, or excessive load-bearing stress—whether or not clinical symptoms of herniation and disk disease are present. Once established, this reduction in disk volume and intervertebral space must invariably alter the mechanics of the posterior spinal segment. A critical change that follows this intervertebral compression is subluxation—an overlap or posterior overriding of the articular processes of the dorsal vertebral arch on either side—at the same vertebral level as the diminution in disk space. Subluxation develops because the functional spinal segment acts as an integral unit and is compressed as a unit; dissociation takes place only in the advent of a fracture at the dorsal vertebral arch with spondylolisthesis. Moreover, at the affected vertebral level, there is a concommitant dorsal displacement of the upper spinal segment with a dorsal shift in the center of rotation; this results in both a loss of lordosis at rest and a reduction in the extent of flexion and extension at that level. The limits of pain-free movement

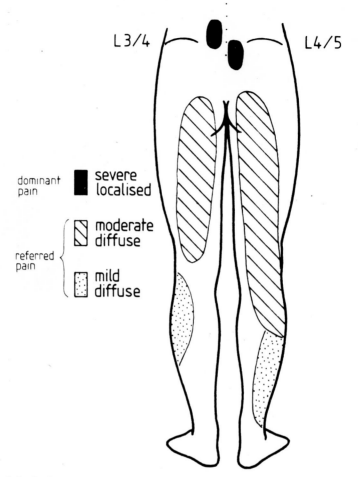

FIG. 3. Pain distribution in facet syndrome. Referred pain patterns from facet joints reflect the distribution of the segmental nerve supply at each level involved. Distal reference to the buttocks relates to the caudad migration of posterior branches, whereas limb distribution mimicking root pain results from pain reference in the anterior division of each segmental nerve.

are thereby reduced, imposing additional demand on adjacent vertebral levels for any further mobility. Consequent to this, or following surgical disk removal or spinal fusion, the adjacent vertebral joints show an increased rate of the same degenerative change so that the disorder tends to progress steadily in a cephalad direction within the spinal column.

With mechanical dysfunction and facet overlap causing impingement on non-articular bony surfaces at upper and lower extremes of the facet joint, capsular irritation and local inflammation ensue. In the acute exacerbation, this causes acute pain, reflex spasm of the posterior erector spinae muscles, and a clinical picture of the acute sprung back.

NORMAL ALIGNMENT

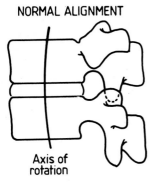

Axis of
rotation

MALALIGNMENT IN DEGENERATIVE
DISEASE

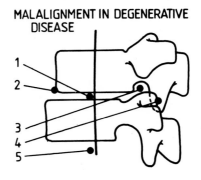

FIG. 4. Skeletal changes in facet syndrome. Dysfunction consequent to degenerative changes. 1. Reduction in intervertebral segment. 2. Backward displacement of vertebral segment. 3. Reduction in aperture size of intervertebral foramen. 4. Subluxation of facet processes, leading to osteophytic growth. 5. Displacement and restriction of vertebral rotation—the fixed erect spine.

In time, several other consequences ensue from this process of facet overriding. Chronic irritation at the articular margins leads to new bone formation and the production of osteophytes that may further limit the range of pain-free movement. The intervertebral foramen that conducts the segmental spinal nerves and vessels becomes progressively narrowed as the intervertebral space diminishes, and further encroachment by osteophytic outgrowths can markedly reduce foraminal size to the point of causing functional stenosis and root pain. Advanced degenerative cases may show both facet and root pain and even spinal stenosis as a result of this progression of events at the one segmental level. This clinical picture may manifest with acute exacerbations, especially with minor traumatic events, or may be present as an unremitting chronic diffuse pain. Specific lesions related to disk prolapse are separate entities but may also present concurrently with this spondylosis.

CLINICAL PRESENTATION

As with most disorders of the vertebral column and its integuments, there is no singular feature or set of symptoms and signs that confers an absolute diagnosis of facet joint disease. A compilation of the major features will, however, give a composite presentation for most of the cases that are likely to be encountered.

1. Dominant pain is seen around the lower lumbar or lumbosacral levels, usually aching in quality.

2. Diffuse, lesser intensity, referred pains are present over buttocks and posterolateral thigh, occasionally extending to the lateral calf level (see Fig. 3).

3. Pain is aggravated with sustained posture, especially standing or sitting. Driving a vehicle is a common factor. Sudden movements, jarring, load carrying, hyperextension are common causes of acute exacerbation or aggravation.

4. Relief can be obtained with rest and local heat application. Some reduction of pain may result if the patient holds the spine in a slightly flexed neutral position.

5. The spine is held fairly rigid during walking with a loss of lordosis and a reduction in spinal mobility at the affected level. Loss of "springing" can be affirmed at the involved segment.

6. Mild to moderate tenderness is found along the paraspinal muscles on the involved side with similar tenderness to palpation over the iliolumbar and sacroiliac ligaments when the lower two lumbar levels are involved.

7. More pronounced, focal tenderness is found on deep palpation over the involved facet joint, when pressure is applied with a thumb or finger through relaxed overlying muscle layers.

8. Neurological changes may be equivocal and inconsistent between successive examinations. Mild sensory, reflex, and motor changes are encountered, possibly reflecting referred phenomena in those segmental nerves subserving nociceptive input from the involved joints.

9. Straight leg raising is usually restricted by pain and tightness in the back and/or the hamstrings. Lack of further pain with dorsiflexion of the foot is critical in distinguishing a facet syndrome pain from that caused by root irritation.

10. The correlation between radiological changes and clinical symptoms is surprisingly poor. Extensive disk space reduction and degenerative bony changes do not necessarily relate to pain intensity, and some patients with acute pain show no bony abnormality. Nevertheless, each patient should have one set of X-rays taken to exclude bone pathology.

11. The final and ultimate confirmation of facet joint disease is obtained by injection of local anaesthetic into the joint or its nerve supply. Abolition of pain and tenderness accompanied by some functional improvement virtually ensures the diagnosis.

12. Features of both root pain and facet irritation are often present at the same level in advanced cases. In such situations, therapy may be directed to both entities, providing both an epidural and a facet block in successive treatments.

INDICATIONS FOR FACET BLOCK

Because facet joint disease is essentially chronic, although it may have acute exacerbations, treatment with facet injections should be reserved for those patients who are unresponsive to simpler, noninvasive therapies. Approaches to early management should utilize whatever skills are available to individual practitioners or can be readily obtained from local resources. To this end, a structured acute care program will vary considerably between localities and even between different practitioners. Nevertheless, basic objectives remain the same, namely, to overcome acute episodes rapidly and safely, with the minimum intervention at the least cost, and, in the longer term, to sustain remission and function, minimizing disease progression and frequency of acute attacks. The available options are extensive, but they all encompass the use of one or several of the following in sequence or concurrently, depending on the patient's presentation and the resource's availability.

1. Analgesics. A combined program of anti-inflammatory and centrally acting drugs prescribed to full tolerated doses is appropriate. Transcutaneous electrical stimulation provides an additional reserve analgesia system if needed or may by itself give adequate pain relief for some.

2. Muscle relaxation. Drug-induced reduction of spasm with diazepam or baclofen may be effective in acute attacks, but long-term, muscle-relaxing drugs are not only ineffective but may also induce drug dependence, sleep disturbance, and anxiety/depression. Far more appropriate for the patient with chronic low back pain is a program in relaxation training or biofeedback therapy. Skilled operators in a multidisciplinary setting are essential to get the best results with these techniques; however, their effectiveness is profound and may be the critical element in ultimate functional rehabilitation.

3. Manipulation. This too requires special skills and experience, yielding best results when applied early. In general, the response is not sustained unless the procedure is repeated frequently and combined with other treatments, exercise, and analgesics in particular.

4. Heat and cold. Applications of these assist in breaking reflex muscle spasm and have a pain-relieving action as well.

5. Exercise. The currect practice is to recommend exercise rather than rest so that mobility, function, and strength are maintained once effective pain relief has been achieved. Rest is beneficial during acute phases when the primary treatment objective is to resolve local spasm and inflammation, but if prolonged, rest leads to weakness, dysfunction, and delayed rehabilitation.

If an intensive 2-week program of treatment proves ineffective, as it does in a small group of patients, the next step is to undertake an epidural or facet block depending on the clinical presentation. Often a succession of the two may be appropriate, as shown in Fig. 5.

FACET DENERVATION TECHNIQUES

Several methods have been described, some involving joint denervation, others periarticular or capsular injection. Historically, Rees's technique of surgical percutaneous rhizolysis (10) served to introduce the concept but has been discarded for the safer and more accurate percutaneous needle or probe techniques, which are aided by the use of an X-ray image intensifier.

With the patient lying prone and the back slightly flexed over pillows, the appropriate facet level is marked at the sites of maximum focal tenderness. It is usual to treat between two and four facets on either side at each procedure. At each site, approximately 3 cm lateral to the spinous process towards its lower edge, local anesthetic is infiltrated into the skin and fascial layers and a probe or spinal needle (depending on the technique employed) is advanced to the facet joint under fluoroscopic surveillance. A safe and successful block cannot be consistently obtained without this aid. Diagnostic block as the initial step employs 2 ml of 1% lidocaine at each level to confirm the diagnosis. Definitive treatment may utilize injection of

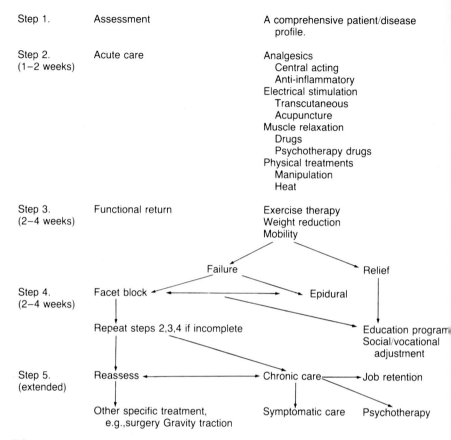

Step 1.   Assessment   A comprehensive patient/disease
                                                       profile.

Step 2.   Acute care   Analgesics
(1–2 weeks)   Central acting
                                                         Anti-inflammatory
                                                       Electrical stimulation
                                                         Transcutaneous
                                                         Acupuncture
                                                       Muscle relaxation
                                                         Drugs
                                                         Psychotherapy drugs
                                                       Physical treatments
                                                         Manipulation
                                                         Heat

Step 3.   Functional return   Exercise therapy
(2–4 weeks)   Weight reduction
                                                       Mobility

Failure   Relief

Step 4.   Facet block ← ──────────→ Epidural
(2–4 weeks)

Repeat steps 2,3,4 if incomplete   Education program
                                                       Social/vocational
                                                       adjustment

Step 5.   Reassess ←──────→ Chronic care ──→ Job retention
(extended)

Other specific treatment,   Symptomatic care   Psychotherapy
e.g.,surgery Gravity traction

FIG. 5.   A schematic flow chart for treatment of acute exacerbations of low back pain.

methyl prednisolone (Depo-Medrol) 20 mg in 2 to 4 ml bupivacaine at each level or use 7% phenol in contrast solutions such as Urograffin or Conray, these latter yielding a graphic record of solution spread on subsequent X-ray. In both instances, the aim is periarticular infiltration of the painful joint, rather than joint denervation. Correct needle placement is determined by the "feel" of its lying within the joint and by fluoroscopy.

Denervation alone, remote from the facet joint, requires even greater precision of needle or probe placement, with both X-ray surveillance and electrical stimulation employed to ensure accuracy. In this case, the probe is more commonly advanced slightly more lateral to the facet process so that it is at the junction of the superior edge of the transverse process and the dorsal lumbar process of the spinal arch. At this level, a small intertransverse ligament can be felt at the limit of needle or probe advancement. Because of the dual origin of joint innervation, lesions must be made at the levels of both the involved joint and the segment just above. In all cases, direct needle or light electrical stimulation, either around the joint itself or at the level of its nerve supply, should simulate the patient's pain in both quality and distribution. X-ray films taken at this time will further confirm accuracy of placement with greater clarity than fluoroscopy and will also serve as a permanent record of the procedure for the patient's file (Fig. 6).

Alternatives available for inducing neurolysis consist of heat lesions produced with a radiofrequency generator, cold lesions with a nitrous oxide cryoprobe, and chemical destruction with phenol solutions. Having utilized surgical, chemical, and cryogenic methods, the authors still find it difficult to state which is superior, although the surgical method is unquestionably inferior in every respect. Neurolytic and steroid injections are probably the easiest, but these solutions tend to spread in narrow linear planes and do not produce the more certain radial lesions seen with destruction by heat or cold. Cold and radiofrequency generators are more cumbersome and expensive and require a greater probe size to produce the lesion. By whatever method, the entire treatment is completed in less than 15 min and can be safely done on an outpatient basis, even when three levels are treated on each side.

Arguments can be expressed in favor of either direct joint injection techniques or denervation procedures proximal to the joint. Regarding articular injections, the greatest advantage is that only one needle approach is needed for each joint and needles can be narrow gauge, producing minimal discomfort for the patient. Whether

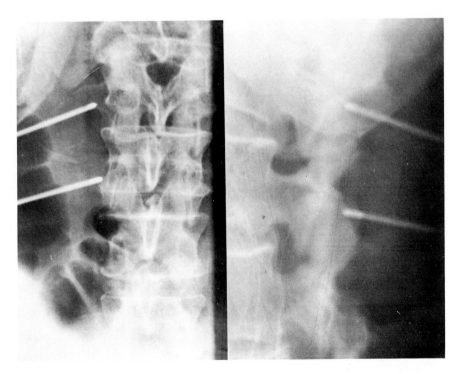

FIG. 6. Positioning of probes for facet denervation. Courtesy of E. G. Richards.

injections at this level act by a neurolytic, sclerosant, or anti-inflammatory action is not apparent, nor can any clinical difference in the response to different solution types be determined. However, in all instances, patients are advised to expect an initial aggravation of pain before the block takes full effect.

Denervation procedures at the posterior primary ramus have a major advantage in that afferent stimuli from all the posterior elements of the spinal column, plus ligaments and soft tissues, will be interrupted. Therefore, nociceptive input from all areas—ligaments, for example—whether separate or secondary to mechanical dysfunction, will be abolished concurrently with input from the joint itself. Such therapy might be useful against wider sources of pain, especially in chronic situations, or when the precise localization of pain within a given spinal segment is difficult.

At our present level of knowledge, it is not clear which technique might have the greatest merit.

CLINICAL GUIDELINES

Practical guidance becomes increasingly difficult as discussion moves from the basic concerns of facet innervation and the pathogenesis of low back pain to the application of facet injection or denervation techniques in the demands of everyday clinical care. Here, the combination of semantic differences and multinational and multidisciplinary variations in approach and the complexity of multifunctional presentations are such that it would be naive to expect a single treatment modality to be uniformly effective. The need is to present not "the cure" but rather something less ambitious. Perhaps, in the light of present limitations, this might be that combination of therapies that yields the best sustained symptomatic and functional relief for each patient. The vagaries of combined skeletal, muscular, and behavior disorders encountered in the entity of facet syndrome pain almost deny the precision of single therapy control, so important in setting up well conducted clinical studies. Neither is there sufficient consistency in assessment, treatment, and follow-up to meet the needs and logistics of undertaking multicenter trials. Rothman's Pennsylvania Plan (11) and other similar algorithms will assist considerably in improving care for individual patients and advancing collective experience. The advent of readily available computerization of vast data variables will also enhance our ability to conduct future trials. However, the current need is to evolve a program on the basis of available methods and results. To this end, a therapeutic sequence is provided, with the realization that it is neither all inclusive nor detailed in the provision of each aspect of care—although most if not all options are covered by other chapters in this volume. The plan is not necessarily specific to facet syndrome pain nor is it applicable to low back pain other than that caused by readily recognizable specific pathological states.

What remains essential to this approach is the need to set up a working diagnosis, with a treatment plan followed by early assessment. According to the degree of response or remaining impairment, subsequent or concurrent therapy is instituted until failure or success determines entry into alternative or further steps. The overriding principle remains one of symptomatic and functional relief—an important distinction from that of cure and one that needs to be explained to the patient in promoting long-term management strategy. In the treatment plan shown in Fig. 5, the availability of local resources will determine the particular skills and sequences to be used. For any patient, the entry level for each of the treatment options will clearly differ according to the patient's presentation and local resources. From a management standpoint, it should be stressed that the treatment options may be provided concurrently, that failure of one option does not preclude trial with another within the same area of treatment, and that disorders involving the sacroiliac point or soft tissues may arise either separately or consequent to facet pain and will require further treatment in their own right.

Surgery, although included in the flow chart, has virtually no place in treatment of facet syndrome pain itself but may be necessary in the presence of instability associated with spondylolisthesis or when there is disk prolapse or stenotic cord or root compression.

For its own part, disk surgery may accentuate the development of interlaminar subluxation by reducing the intervertebral space, thus further increasing facetal overlap. Facet injections are especially successful under these circumstances but are less appropriate for other postsurgical causes of low back pain such as soft tissue scarring or entrapment, nerve damage, or vascular pain (1,2).

A serious contention concerns who best should undertake facet denervation techniques. It probably does not matter, but the ever-present medical dictum that one physician should take total clinical responsibility for the patient, while altruistic and professionally desirable, may not always be in the patient's best interest. Like surgery, facet injections, nerve blocks, epidurals, etc. are probably done best by technical experts, whereas continuing care and patient management is best undertaken by a primary physician or a medical orthopedist. When supervised in this manner, a patient is more likely to proceed to appropriate treatments quickly, without the limitations and delays of being caught within the restrictions of a narrow singular specialty interest. Unfortunately, so overwhelming is the need for treatment in the community at large, that almost any legitimate practitioner from any discipline can establish a busy practice on the basis of one or a narrow group of treatment modalities. Clearly the medicosocial implications demand a better trained specialist in musculoskeletal medicine, one not bound by past traditions but equipped to deal with probably all but the surgical requirements of this ever-increasing field.

RESULTS

As stated, the disappointing aspect of facet denervation treatment remains the paucity of controlled long-term trials. For the present, in the absence of uniformly accepted criteria for entry, technique, and follow-up assessment, patient responses can be graded only in terms of symptomatic and functional change. In the several clinical reports to date, most authors quote a success rate of 60% or more of their patients gaining a good sustained improvement following treatment. Some 400 patients in our own experience have a similar good response rate, though the use of neurolytic injections, introduced in 1974 after high morbidity and failure with the Rees technique, was in turn superceded by steroid rather than phenol injections. Results with phenol were good, resembling those reported by Hickey and Tregonning (5); the subsequent Depo-Medral injections also gave favorable results, similar to those described by Mooney and Robertson (9). There seemed little difference between our two treatments, but more recently a trial with cryotherapy has been initiated by E. G. Richards in our clinic, on the basis of the technique developed by Lloyd et al. (6). Although initial results are promising, the undoubted improvement in diagnosis and ancillary therapy with several years experience makes any intergroup comparison dubious.

The best publicized study to date is that of Mehta and Sluijter (8), who showed that approximately 50% of their patients did well on initial evaluation but that at 1-year follow-up, half of those initially successful cases had relapsed. In their study, which employed well-controlled clinical, therapeutic, and evaluation criteria, a radiofrequency-induced heat lesion was used as the denervation treatment. Whether further refinements of technique can improve on their results is the challenge for all. Perhaps the saving factor in this procedure is that the morbidity level is almost zero, with no serious sequelae yet reported in this or other studies. Notwithstanding these somewhat disappointing long-term results is the fact that all these patients had truly chronic conditions, totally unresolved by previous treatments, and were therefore burdened with continuing pain and disability but for the intervention of a facet block. Viewed in this context, any treatment that yields a 30 to 50% success rate must be viewed as a considerable advance. The further improvement up to 80% gained from including multispecialty treatment such as psychotherapy, physical treatments, drug supervision, and vocational retraining ensures that even fewer patients enter the specter of chronic disabling low back pain.

CONCLUSIONS

Despite the concerns that have been expressed, recognition of the facet syndrome as a major cause of chronic low back pain has focused attention on the posterior laminar elements of the spine as a site for investigation and treatment. On current evidence, the concept of treatment with facet joint injections or denervation appears to be sound, based on disruption of functional integrity at the intervertebral/interlaminar level as the primary defect. The technique of facet block is simple, quick, and safe, with virtually no serious consequences, and is therefore appropriate as an outpatient treatment, albeit in a well-equipped clinic or hospital setting. Given these considerations, the results published suggest that the technique warrants more widespread use and further comparison studies. A less well-recognized advantage is that almost any medical practitioner has the capacity to undertake these injection techniques with a minimum of basic training. This gives a still further powerful option for treatment at an early stage, an important factor in breaking recurrent exacerbations and limiting physical and psychological impairment. We await the results of serious long-term studies.

REFERENCES

1. Boas, R. A. (1980): Post surgical low back pain. In: *Problems in Pain*, edited by C. Peck and M. Wallace, pp. 188–191. Pergamon Press, Sydney.
2. Boas, R. A., Berg, D. J., and Shahnarian, A. (1978): Post laminectomy epidural venous changes in chronic low back pain. In: *Second World Congress on Pain, Vol. 1.*, Abstracts, p. 248. International Association for the Study of Pain. Seattle.
3. Bradley, K. C. (1974): The anatomy of backache. *Aust. N. Z. J. Surg.*, 44:227–232.
4. Edgar, M. A., and Ghadially, J. A. (1976): Innervation of the lumbar spine. *Clin. Orthop.*, 115:35–41.
5. Hickey, R. F. J., and Tregonning, G. D. (1977): Denervation of spinal facet joints for treatment of chronic low back pain. *N. Z. Med. J.*, 85:96–99.
6. Lloyd, J. W., Barnard, J. D. W., and Glynn, C. J. (1976): Cryoanalgesia, a new approach to pain relief. *Lancet*, 2:932–934.
7. MacNab, I. (1977): *Backache*. Williams & Wilkins, Baltimore.
8. Mehta, M., and Sluijter, M. E. (1979): The treatment of chronic back pain. *Anaesthesia*, 34:768–775.
9. Mooney, V., and Robertson, J. (1976): The facet syndrome. *Clin. Orthop.*, 115:149–156.
10. Rees, W. E. S. (1971): Multiple bilateral subcutaneous rhizolysis of segmental nerves in the treatment of the inter-vertebral disc syndrome. *Ann. Gen. Prac.*, 26:126–127.
11. Rothman, R. H., and Holmes, H. E. (1979): The Pennsylvania plan: An algorithm for the management of lumbar degenerative disc disease. In: *Advances in Pain and Therapy, Vol. 3*, edited by J. J. Bonica, J. C. Liebeskind, and D. G. Albe-Fessard. Raven Press, New York.
12. Shealy, C. N. (1975): Percutaneous radiofrequency denervation of spinal facets. *J. Neurosurg.*, 43:448–451.

Chronic Low Back Pain, edited by
M. Stanton-Hicks and Robert Boas.
Raven Press, New York © 1982.

Unconventional Approaches: Chymopapain and Alternative Neurosurgical Techniques

Harold A. Wilkinson

*Department of Neurosurgery, University of Massachusetts Medical Center,
Worcester, Massachusetts 01605*

Chronic back pain is a problem of great magnitude in terms of both the number of people that it affects and its capacity for disrupting lives. Because the conventional solutions so often fail, we must look imaginatively at the problem and consider unconventional approaches (8).

The first of these unconventional neurosurgical approaches to be considered is *prevention of surgery*. Finneson, in his book on low back pain (3), describes this very nicely when he states: "Probably the most common cause of surgical failure is an error of judgment with regard to the indication for initial surgery." Calabro and Berg (see Chapters 4 and 7, *this volume*) have enumerated multiple causes of back disease in addition to lumbar disk rupture, and yet it is very discouraging to find in talking about back pain to neurosurgeons and orthopedists across the country that many have an almost knee-jerk reaction to patients with back and leg pain: "If the patient has pain, operate!" However, I should qualify this first unconventional dictum with the proviso that sometimes the most conservative approach to a patient *is* early surgical intervention. Surgery is the appropriate solution for an obvious

TABLE 1. *Noninvasive therapy for "failed disk syndrome"*

Exercises
Bed rest
Heat, liniment
Massage
Diathermy or ultrasound
Whirlpool bath
Surface cooling
Analgesics, muscle relaxants
Anti-inflammatory drugs
Pelvic traction
Corset or brace
Manipulation under anesthesia
Transcutaneous neurostimulation, acupuncture
Reassurance and support
Psychotherapy

and surgically correctable problem that does not respond rapidly or adequately to nonsurgical therapy. In other words, don't let your patient develop a chronic pain neurosis.

One should use a systematic approach to all patients with back and leg pain, both those that have not undergone previous surgery and those who suffer from the "failed disk syndrome"—which, of course, should really be entitled the "failed disk-operation syndrome." The list of potential therapies is long. Noninvasive therapies (Table 1) have been discussed in other chapters. I would emphasize one of these unconventional, noninvasive neurosurgical approaches: reassurance and support. Few busy neurosurgeons have time for this. The patient's knowledge that he or she has been carefully examined and evaluated and that nothing serious has been discovered frequently encourages him or her to resume functioning in spite of modest residual pain. It is always more reassuring to tell a patient that "nothing needs to be done" than to say that "nothing can be done." For some patients such simple reassurance, perhaps reinforced through a series of office visits, may be of utmost importance and may deter them from insisting on seeking increasingly desperate and more radical invasive therapy for a condition that might have improved in time with less involved and less hazardous treatment. I would add to the list of noninvasive therapies in Table 1 osteopathic manipulation, antidepressant and antineuralgic drugs, including phenytoin, carbamazepine, clonazepam, thiamine, and even nicotinic acid. It is worth keeping in mind that chronic pain sufferers also have episodes of acute nociceptive pain requiring short-term muscle relaxant and analgesic medications or other noninvasive therapy.

Needle therapy (Table 2) is especially important if one accepts the additional unconventional neurosurgical postulate that all back pain is not caused by disk disease. One such condition, which is easily treated but often misdiagnosed, is referred to candidly in the published title of an article as "Ischio-gluteal Bursitis—

TABLE 2. *Therapy involving injections for "failed disk syndrome"*

Analgesic and corticosteroid injection of painful sites
  "Trigger points"
  Ligamentous strains
  Arthritic facet joints
  Pseudarthroses
Epidural corticosteroid injection of nerve roots
Intradiskal corticosteroid injection
Facet nerve blocks
  Anesthetic injection
  Phenol injection
  Radiofrequency nerve block
Intrathecal injections
  Corticosteroids
  Iced and/or hypertonic saline
  Alcohol or phenol

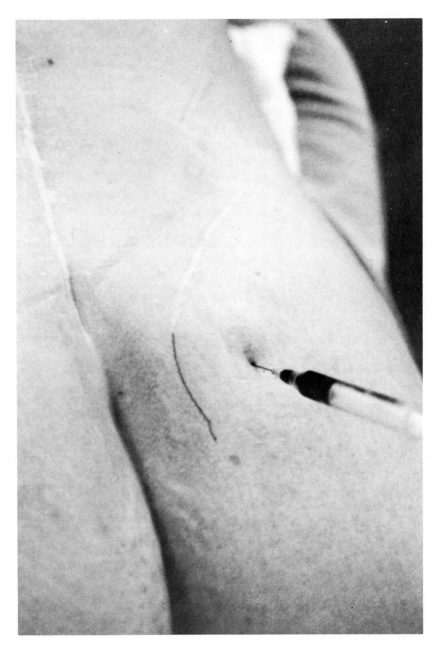

FIG. 1. "Prolotherapy" injection of painful bone-graft donor site in a patient who had experienced excellent but short-lived pain relief from several previous local injections of depository corticosteroids.

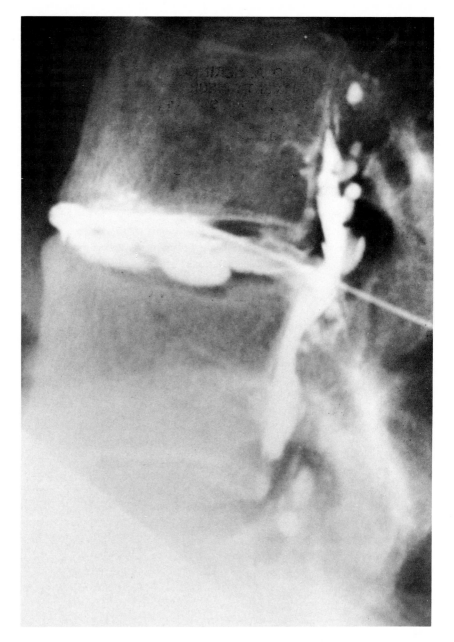

FIG. 2. Abnormal diskogram with posterior extravasation of dye following posterolateral disk injection in a patient with a normal myelogram but surgically proven free disk fragment at operative exploration.

The Classical Pain in the Arse" (7). Depository corticosteroids injected directly into lumbar and lumbosacral trigger points are often beneficial. But what does one do with a patient who consistently attains excellent relief that lasts only 4 to 8 weeks? How many steroid injections can safely be given at any one site? An alternative to consider is "prolotherapy." I am not a member of the National Prolotherapy Society, even though there is one. Injecting a solution of phenol in glycerol and bupivacaine hydrochloride is said to strengthen ligaments at the site of injection, but in my opinion, it is equally likely to be effective because of the neurolytic action of phenol. Nonetheless, this solution can apparently be injected repeatedly in the same site with relative impunity, including in a bone-graft donor site (Fig. 1) or a painful "trigger site."

Diskography can be a valuable diagnostic and therapeutic tool for the neurosurgeon. The classic disk-rupture pattern seen on the diskogram in Fig. 2 belongs to a patient who had a normal myelogram but was found to have a free fragment on surgical exploration. The combination of anesthesia diskography and contrast diskography often materially improves diagnostic accuracy, especially in patients whose pain is predominantly in the back. In many patients with disk degeneration visible on diskography, the severe back pain can be reproduced by injecting the disk under local anesthesia—and all diskograms should be done under local anesthesia if they are to have any meaningful value. If anesthetizing the disk then temporarily relieves the patient of back pain, therapy that is specifically directed at that disk is more likely to succeed.

Such patients may ultimately prove to be ideal candidates for chymopapain injections. In the United States 17,000 patients were injected with chymopapain in a nonrandomized clinical trial (6); results indicated a 68% rate of success in relieving patients of back pain, with two deaths and a 3% rate of anaphylactic reactions. Subsequently, in a double-blind, randomized comparison of chymopapain versus the cysteine-edetate-iothalamate (CEI) carrier solution in 104 patients (1), no statistically significant difference in improvement rate between the two groups was found; 58% of the chymopapain group showed improvement compared with 50% in the CEI control group, a difference that was only slightly higher than the expected placebo effect. These findings have been challenged, and it has been pointed out that a 1-year follow-up has shown a higher percentage of persistent good results with chymopapain (5). Nonetheless, the study convinced the FDA to declare a moratorium on further clinical study of chymopapain in the United States.

Currently, with FDA approval, a triple-blind study is underway in eight centers across the United States—one is the University of Massachusetts Medical Center— in which intradiskal injections of chymopapain, carrier solution, and saline are compared. The entry criteria are extremely rigid; patients may be accepted only if they present with a classic lumbar disk rupture picture, have pain of greater intensity in the legs than in the back, have objective abnormalities on examination, and have an abnormal myelogram or epidural venogram. Because of the tight restrictions, only 12 patients have been treated in the eight centers in the first 4 months of this

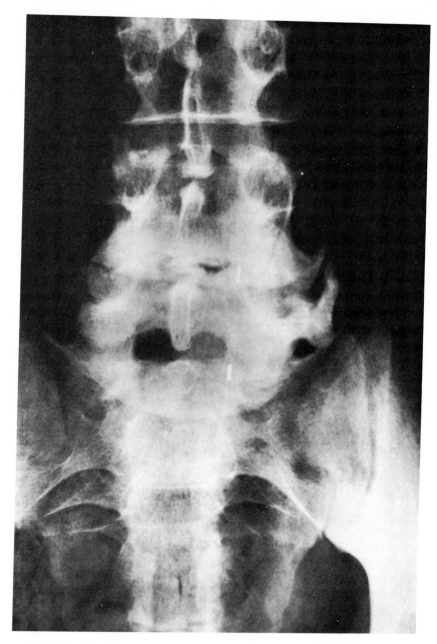

FIG. 3. Severe focal degenerative arthritic changes occurring at the site of a previous two-level disk excision (at the level of metal marking clips) with later development of back pain that remained chronically severe.

TABLE 3. *Surgical therapy for "failed disk syndrome"*

Repeat laminectomy or revision of fusion
Spinal fusion
Facet nerve interruption
Sensory rhizotomy
Anterolateral spinal cordotomy
Prefrontal leukotomy, cingulotomy

study. Four of those were treated here. So far, we do not know which injection they received, but all four showed improvement.

An alternative to intradiskal injection with chymopapain is currently available, and that is intradiskal injection of long-acting corticosteroids. In 1969, Feffer reported a 4- to 10-year follow-up of 244 patients who were given single injections of 25 mg of hydrocortisone mixed with 1.5 ml of Diodrast or Hypaque into two or more interspaces (1). His patients included both those with objective neurologic loss and those with back pain alone. In 67% of his patients, remission occurred either immediately or within 48 hr, and 47% maintained their remission for at least 1 year. He concluded that this procedure was most successful in older patients with predominantly subacute back pain whose plain X-rays and diskograms showed only limited degenerative changes of the involved interspace.

Two years ago, I reviewed my own series of 29 patients with lumbar pain and 13 patients with cervical pain who were treated with intradiskal injections of long-acting steroids (9). The patients were generally selected for this form of treatment only if they were considered not to be obviously good surgical candidates. Accordingly, myelograms were abnormal in only 21% of the lumbar group, although 75% showed some degenerative changes on plain films of the spine. Abnormalities were demonstrated on diskograms in all patients prior to the intradiskal steroid injections. In this group of problem patients, 54% achieved a good result, defined as significant pain improvement lasting a minimum of 3 months. In agreement with Feffer's observations, results were better in those patients with predominately diskogenic, or back, pain.

Surgical intervention (Table 3) is appropriately placed in the third or last category of therapies for patients who either have the "failed disk syndrome" or have not undergone an operation. This is not to suggest that patients should be denied appropriate surgery but is intended to emphasize careful patient selection. The minimum prerequisite for surgery should be the demonstration or strong clinical suspicion of a surgically correctable, organic lesion. With this prerequisite established, I personally consider there to be two indications for back surgery. The first is *progressive* neurologic deficit. The presence simply of sensory loss, reflex loss, or mild motor weakness does not necessitate urgent surgical intervention, since many of these neurologic deficits will clear with nonsurgical therapy. However, a progressive loss of neurologic function or severe loss that does not clear rapidly

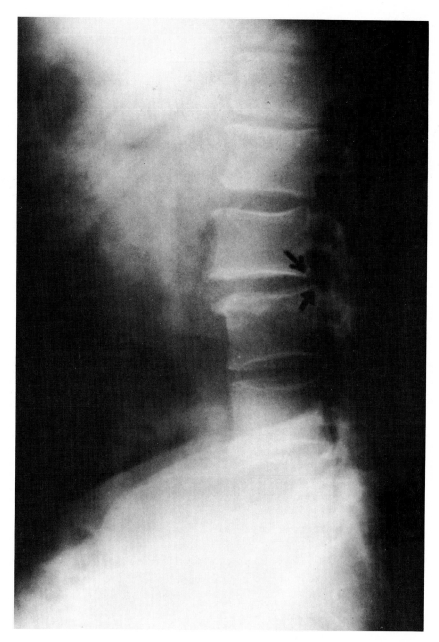

FIG. 4. Spondylolisthesis *(arrows)* noted a decade following spinal fusion from L4 to sacrum with later development of back pain that became chronic.

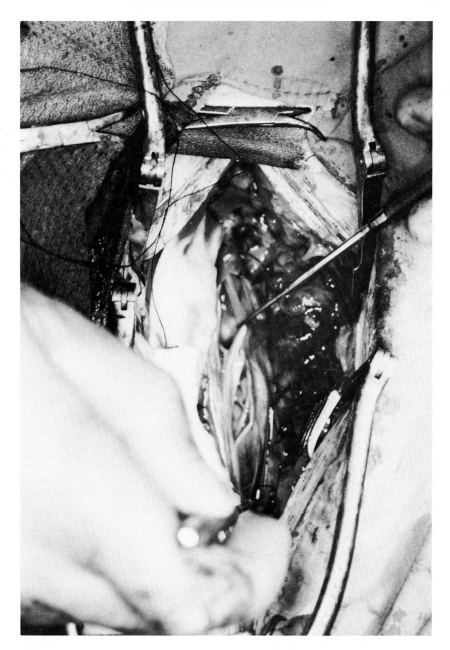

FIG. 5. Lumbar sensory rhizotomy performed for chronic sciatic pain. Motor rootlet is being elevated on the instrument that enters the field from above after the sensory rootlet has been cut with the microscissors in the operator's right hand. Metal clips can be seen attached to distal ends of two sensory roots.

should definitely call for surgery. The second indication for surgery is intolerable pain. This obviously introduces a significant element of philosophy, since pain may be intolerable because of its high intensity despite a brief duration; it may be intolerable because of very prolonged duration despite moderate intensity; or it may be intolerable because of multiple relapses, which by their frequency become intolerable.

The question of when to reexplore a lumbar laminectomy performed by another surgeon is a particularly difficult one. To operate on the premise that the other surgeon's operation was insufficient is fraught with danger, not only of failure but also of actually making the patient worse. Many surgeons would disagree with me but I believe that a previous failure from back surgery is not in itself an indication for an operation. There are, however, many documented cases of an inadequate initial surgical exploration, especially in conditions such as lateral recess stenosis or retained disk fragments.

Adding a back fusion to a previously unsuccessful simple diskectomy can be either gratifying or frustrating. Figure 3 shows severe arthritic changes that developed 15 years later in a patient who did not have a back fusion. However, in the patient whose X-ray is shown in Fig. 4, spondylothesis developed above the fusion, resulting in severe back pain. If relief is obtained from external bracing, more optimism is warranted. Pseudoarthrosis of a previous fusion is a particularly difficult problem, since X-rays, even laminograms and bending films, are usually inconclusive. Pseudoarthrosis does predominantly cause back pain, but the underlying dense epidural scar can include nerve roots as well, so that repair of pseudoarthrosis with epidural neurolysis may improve both radicular and lumbar pain components.

Chordotomy, performed either by open surgery or by percutaneous technique, is rarely, if ever, indicated or successful in the patient with failed disk syndrome. For the patient whose pain is predominantly radicular, sensory rhizotomy at one or two roots may be quite valuable (Fig. 5). The literature varies widely on this subject, with success rates ranging from 75% to as low as 25%. My own experience falls halfway between and includes a number of patients who have been restored to gainful occupations after years of painful disability.

Psychosurgical methods such as prefrontal leukotomy should never be employed for the "failed disk syndrome" alone but on rare occasions may be useful for pain relief in patients with severe psychiatric disorders complicated by this syndrome. It should always be borne in mind that suicide is one of the recognized complications of the failed back syndrome. Stereotactic cingulotomy (Fig. 6) has been recommended for chronic back sufferers who are severely anxious or depressed because of their pain. In 1973, Hurt and Ballantine reported on the Massachusetts General Hospital experience with 68 patients who underwent cingulotomy for intractable pain (4). Of these, 36 patients suffered from nonmalignant conditions—8 of them patients with a failed disk syndrome—and 32 had carcinomas. Pain relief was found to be better in patients with chronic fixed pain than in those with cancer. Thus, in the former group, 23% experienced marked to complete relief of pain, 44% experienced slight to moderate relief, and 33% had no relief. My own more limited

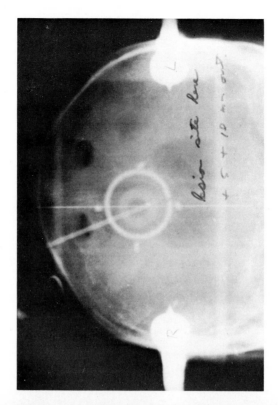

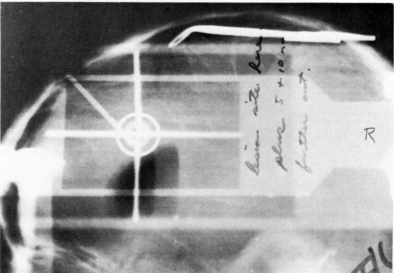

FIG. 6. Stereotactic cingulotomy performed for intractable pain in a suicidally depressed patient with "failed back syndrome." A radiofrequency probe is placed in the cingulate gyrus to produce a bilateral lesion. Front view *(top)* and lateral view *(bottom)* of skull showing limited ventriculogram and stereotactic guides directing the radiofrequency probe to its target.

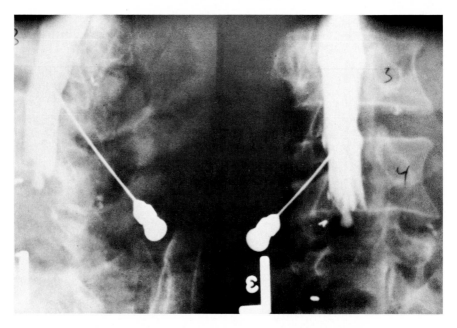

FIG. 7. Complete transverse adhesive arachnoiditis in a patient who had previously undergone disk excision at two levels. The multiple-level disk excision raises the possibility that, in fact, neither disk was truly ruptured but that the underlying disease might have been primary arachnoiditis.

results likewise suggest that most patients will receive some benefit from this surgery, although I have not yet encountered a patient who obtained complete relief from pain, and in some the pain relief is limited indeed. The effects of the stereotactic cingulate gyrus lesions are quite interesting; these lesions seem to interrupt the self-propagating flywheel of suffering, which is presumably kept alive in the limbic circuitry of the brain. As a result, the patient's level of suffering gradually subsides over a period of weeks or a few months after surgery, and relief is likely to be maintained unless a new source of pain arises. It is for this reason that cancer patients achieve such limited results. The procedure causes no detectable intellectual impairment, and in fact the President's Commission on Psychosurgery reported that the only consistent change in measurable mental status in postoperative IQ testing was a slight *improvement* in performance—attributed to less distraction from suffering and smaller intake of medication.

The last disorder to be discussed in this chapter is lumbar adhesive arachnoiditis. Approximately 250,000 lumbar laminectomies are performed annually in the United States, and it is estimated that 10 to 40% of these end in the failed disk syndrome. Many of these patients develop some form of arachnoiditis—a protean condition varying from simple nerve-root blunting to complete transverse obliteration of the lumbar thecal sac (Fig. 7). Patients with this disorder may remain asymptomatic,

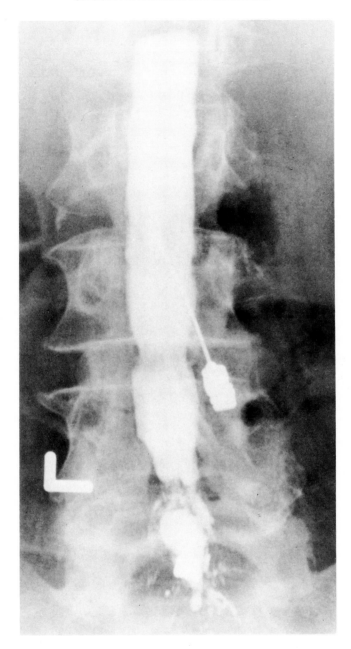

FIG. 8. Complete transverse adhesive arachnoiditis at L4/5 in an asymptomatic patient who underwent myelography for cervical disease. Note two lumbar puncture needles, one partially obscured at L5/S1.

TABLE 4. *Preoperative symptoms and signs of patients with arachnoiditis*

Symptoms and signs	Total (%)	Unilateral	Bilateral
Severe pain[a]	17 (100)	8	9
Sensory loss	14 (82)	7	7
Motor weakness	7 (41)	4	3
Bladder symptoms	3 (18)	—	—
Bowel impairment	1 (6)	—	—

[a]Only symptom in three patients.

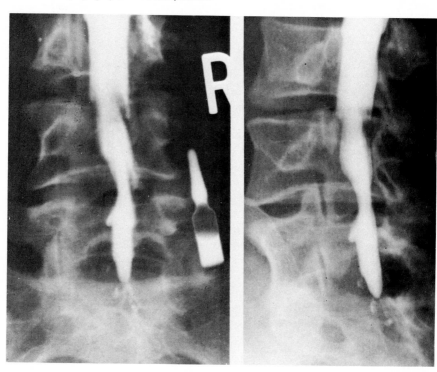

FIG. 9. Myelogram interpreted as showing a large disk rupture at L4/5 in a patient who subsequently developed adhesive arachnoiditis. Surgical exploration failed to confirm a frank disk rupture but intradural exploration was not carried out.

back surgery. In the myelogram of her back (Fig. 8), a needle was first placed at L5/S1, and there was a complete block to Pantopaque; a second needle, placed at L2/3, demonstrated a transverse block at L4/5, a totally asymptomatic area. However, most of these patients suffer pain and variable neurologic deficits, which may at times be progressive. Even asymptomatic forms of arachnoiditis can cause problems, since they may obscure surgically correctable lesions and deter surgeons from otherwise beneficial operative intervention.

TABLE 5. *Results of operation for arachnoiditis*

Result	Length of follow-up	
	< 1 yr	> 1 yr
Decreased pain		
Poor relief	4/17	[a]6/12
Fair relief	7/17 ⎫ 13/17 (76%)	3/12 ⎫ 6/12 (50%)
Good/excellent relief	6/17 ⎭	3/12 ⎭
Neurological improvement		
Sensory loss	10/14 ⎫	5/11 ⎫
Motor weakness	1/7 ⎬ 10/14 (71%)	1/6 ⎬ 5/11 (45%)
Bladder/bowel impairment	2/3 ⎭	1/3 ⎭
Neurological worsening		
Sensory loss	2/17 ⎫	1/12 ⎫
Hyperpathia	2/17 ⎬ 3/17 (18%)	0/12 ⎬ 2/12 (17%)
Motor weakness	0/17	[b]1/12
Bladder weakness	1/17 ⎭	[b]1/12 ⎭

[a]Recurrences of pain began 2 months to 5 years after lysis.
[b]One patient was neurologically worse after later rhizotomy.

The etiology of arachnoiditis is obscure. Every series includes examples of spontaneously occurring arachnoiditis, and familial forms have also been reported. Myelography has been implicated as a cause, but this is unlikely for several reasons: (a) arachnoiditis has been seen not only after Pantopaque injection but also following instillation of some of the water-soluble contrast materials; (b) arachnoiditis is rarely, if ever, seen after myelograms done purely for cervical or thoracic disease; (c) arachnoiditis rarely involves either the caudal sac where the Pantopaque should have settled or the needle puncture site where the Pantopaque was introduced; and (d) arachnoiditis is nearly always seen at the level of the "disk disease." Lumbar surgery itself has also been implicated as an etiologic factor. Multiple-level or bilateral surgery prior to discovery of arachnoiditis is common, but that often means simply that extradural findings were equivocal at the first operation. Many patients have had multiple operations before developing arachnoiditis, but others have not.

It is my contention that arachnoiditis is often misdiagnosed initially as lumbar disk disease, and that it occurs as a spontaneous condition. The reason for this contention is that all the patients in my series had bilateral or multiple defects on myelography prior to their first surgical procedures, rather than the typical anterolateral defects seen with disk ruptures; and some of the patients who showed large defects on myelography and limited extradural findings subsequently developed progressive arachnoiditis. If my contention is correct, every surgeon should be aware of this possibility and should be prepared to explore the intradural space if the myelogram demonstrates a large defect but the extradural findings are unimpressive. I might add that I have explored many patients with the "failed back syndrome", and I have not seen the excessive vascularity described by Boas *(this volume)*.

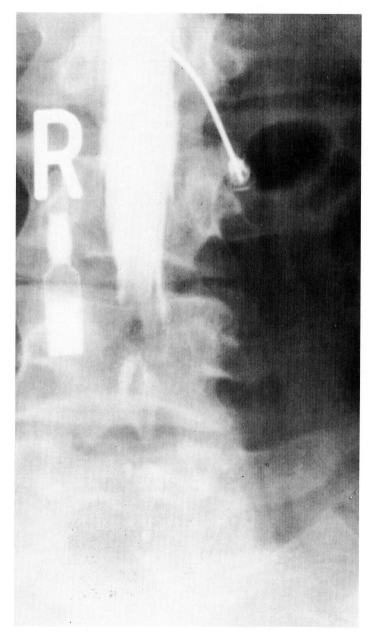

FIG. 10. Myelogram demonstrating complete transverse arachnoiditis at the level of previous diskectomy in the same patient illustrated in Fig. 9.

The myelogram in Fig. 9 was thought to demonstrate a ruptured lumbar disk and the patient underwent surgery. The operative notes which I obtained stated that there was gross bulging in the disk, but it was removed nonetheless. The patient returned with a progressive "failed back syndrome" and now had a transverse defect on the myelogram, typical of adhesive arachnoiditis (Fig. 10).

I have reserved surgical lysis of arachnoiditis for patients disabled by severe pain or severe neurologic deficit that is unresponsive to prolonged nonoperative therapy. In my group of 17 patients (10), 16 had undergone previous surgery or intrumentation, and there was one case of proven spontaneous arachnoitis. All of these patients suffered severe, usually bilateral pain, and 80% exhibited significant neurologic deficits, including three with cauda syndrome (Table 4). Arachnoiditis was demonstrated by loculated Pantopaque in three patients. On myelography a complete transverse block was found in all but one patient. In only five patients did the arachnoidal thickening involve more than one spine level, that of the previous "disk disease"—I use quotes because I question the accuracy of the original diagnosis. One of these five who had a more extensive disease was a patient with spontaneously occurring arachnoiditis and no history of previous instrumentation or surgery.

Microsurgical decompressive surgery was performed in all 17 patients, and each received steroids intrathecally, systemically, or both—during and after surgery. A total of 76% of these patients achieved significant pain relief within the first few months after surgery, and 71% showed objective neurologic improvement (Table 5). By the end of 1 year, the results had deteriorated so that only 50% continued to enjoy pain relief and 45% persistent neurologic improvement. Four of the five patients who were followed for longer than 5 years have maintained their improvement, with one experiencing a slow deterioration that occurred after re-injury following an automobile accident.

In summary, microsurgical intervention for this group of severely afflicted patients disabled by arachnoiditis offers to many, but certainly not all, the chance of some amelioration of their long-standing disabilities.

REFERENCES

1. Cloud, G. A., Doyle, J. E., et al. (1976): *Final Statistical Analysis of the Disease Double Blind Clinical Trial*. Biostatistical Services Dept., Travenol Laboratories, Inc. Dunfall, Ill.
2. Feffer, H. L. (1975): Regional use of steroids in the management of lumbar intervertebral disc disease. *Orthop. Clin. N. Am.*, 6:249–253
3. Finneson, B. E. (1973): *Low Back Pain*. J. B. Lippincott Co., Philadelphia.
4. Hurt, R. W., and Ballantine, H. T., Jr. (1974): Stereotactic anterior cingulate lesions for persistent pain; a report on 68 cases. *Clinical Neurosurgery, Vol. 21*, edited by R. H. Wilkins, pp. 334–351. Williams & Wilkins Co., Baltimore.
5. Martins, A. N., Raminez, A., et al. (1978): Double blind evaluation of chemonucleolysis for herniated lumbar disk: Late results. *J. Neurosurg.*, 49:816–827.
6. Report of the Committee on Chemopapain (Disease). (1974): Chicago, American Academy of Orthopedic Surgeons.
7. Swartout, R., and Compere, E. L. (1974): Ischio-gluteal bursitis: The pain in the arse. *J. A. M. A.*, 227:557–552.
8. Wilkinson, H. A. (1978): Failed disk syndrome. *Family Physician*, 17:86–94.

9. Wilkinson, H. A., and Schuman, N. (1980): Intradiscal corticosteroids in the treatment of lumbar and cervical disc problems. *Spine*, 5:385–389.
10. Wilkinson, H. A., and Schuman, N. (1979): Results of surgical lysis of lumbar adhesive arachnoiditis. *Neurosurgery*, 4:401–409.

Subject Index